O P L

OXFORD PSYCHIATRY LIBRARY

Schizophrenia and Psychiatric Comorbidities

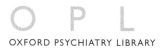

OXFORD PSYCHIATRY LIBRARY

Schizophrenia and Psychiatric Comorbidities

Recognition and Management

David J. Castle

Chair of Psychiatry
St Vincent's Hospital, University of Melbourne
Australia

Peter F. Buckley

Dean
Virginia Commonwealth University, School of Medicine
Richmond,
Virginia, USA

Rachel Upthegrove

Professor
Psychiatry and Youth Mental Health
Institute for Mental Health, University of Birmingham, UK

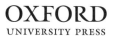
OXFORD
UNIVERSITY PRESS

Great Clarendon Street, Oxford, OX2 6DP,
United Kingdom

Oxford University Press is a department of the University of Oxford.
It furthers the University's objective of excellence in research, scholarship,
and education by publishing worldwide. Oxford is a registered trade mark of
Oxford University Press in the UK and in certain other countries

Published in the United States of America by Oxford University Press
198 Madison Avenue, New York, NY 10016, United States of America

British Library Cataloguing in Publication Data

Data available

Library of Congress Control Number: 2020948005

ISBN 978–0–19–887033–3

DOI: 10.1093/med/9780198870333.001.0001

Printed in Great Britain by
Bell & Bain Ltd., Glasgow

Foreword

This scholarly volume is a very timely and welcome contribution to our field. It addresses and dissects the clinically critical issue of multiple comorbidities in schizophrenia. In addition, it integrates and synthesizes many lines of evidence for the extensive aetiological and clinical overlap among major psychiatric conditions that are currently regarded as free-standing DSM diagnostic categories. The implications for this scholarly scientific review and discourse should ultimately lead to a paradigm shift in conceptualizing the nosology, epidemiology, aetiology, and treatment of major psychiatric disorders including schizophrenia, depression, autism spectrum disorder, attention deficit hyperactivity disorder (ADHD), anxiety, OCD, PTSD and substance use.

For a long time, and prior to the neuroscience revolution that enabled probing the human brain and exploring the neurobiology of psychiatric disorders, the field of psychiatry was descriptive and simplistic. It categorized psychiatric disorders essentially as silos, defined by a set of signs and symptoms. If one or more psychiatric conditions co-occurred with a 'primary diagnosis', they were labelled as 'comorbidities', with no implications of a shared aetiology or biology. Amazingly, despite the rapid accrual of evidence of shared developmental or genetic aetiopathogenesis, dysplasia of the same brain regions on neuroimaging and a shared benefit from the same class of medications, DSM-5 and its traditional out-date schema, remains the diagnostic Bible of Psychiatry.

This archaic model is ripe for change.

The following are highlights of recent advances in re-conceptualizing the nosology of schizophrenia and other DSM diagnostic entities re-interpreting the comorbidities as evidence of the substantial clinical and biological overlap and inter-connectivity of psychiatric brain disorders.

1. Neurodevelopmental Pathology: Disruption of brain development during fetal life has been well established across the schizophrenia syndrome and practically all the so-called comorbidities (Beauchaine et al. 2018; Huttunen and Mednick 2018; Krueger and Eaton 2015).

2. Genetic Pleiotropy: About 50% of the 22,000 protein-coding genes in the human chromosomes are expressed in the brain during development. Schizophrenia and most psychiatric disorders are heavily genetic. Genetic pleiotropy has been identified across several psychiatric syndromes (Nasrallah 2013; Smoller and Cross-Disorder Group of the Psychiatric Genomics Consortium 2019). For example, the calcium channel A1 gene is shared by schizophrenia, autism, bipolar disorder, major depression and ADHD (Gudmundsson et al. 2019). This indicates that the DSM separation of those disorders is artificial and based on specific symptoms without integrating what is regarded as comorbid conditions into a unified model. Copy

number variants have also been found in schizophrenia, ADHD, and autism spectrum disorders (Doernberg and Hollender 2016; Smoller and Cross-Disorder Group of the Psychiatric Genomics Consortium 2019).

3. Neuroimaging Concordance: Three brain regions—the dorsal anterior cingulate, left insula, and right insula—have been reported to be abnormal across schizophrenia, bipolar disorder, major depression, OCD and anxiety. Those shared brain structural abnormalities are associated with various degrees of hypoplasia or atrophy (Goodkind 2015).

4. Intermediate phenotypes have been redefined to accommodate transdiagnostic vulnerabilities and aetiological complexity (Etkin and Cuthbert 2014; Beauchaine and Constantino 2017; Hyman 2019).

5. Shared symptoms have long been observed across various psychiatric disorders, including delusions, hallucinations, depression, anxiety, impulsivity, and autistic and cognitive symptoms (Kessler et al. 2011; Nasrallah 2017, 2019; Grisanzio et al. 2018).

6. Response to Pharmacotherapy: It is well recognized that the same class of psychotropic medications exert therapeutic efficacy across a variety of DSM disorders (Maher and Theodore 2012). The SSRIs and atypical antipsychotic exert efficacy in many psychiatric disorders beyond their original indication, which was approved by the FDA based on a specific DSM diagnosis.

7. Connectomics and neural circuits are now regarded as the neurobiological underpinnings of schizophrenia and other psychiatric disorders, and that may be a key reason for the transdiagnostic overlap (Elliott et al. 2018; Xia et al. 2018; Marshal 2020).

8. Similar neurobiological pathologies have been found to exist in several major psychiatric disorders including neuro-progression, white matter pathology, neuroinflammation, oxidative stress, mitochondrial dysfunction, glutamate pathways disruptions and shortened telomeres (Nasrallah 2017).

9. Familial Clustering: Various psychiatric disorders have been found to have significantly increased odds ratios (OR) among the first-degree relatives of patients with schizophrenia including bipolar 1 (4.27), bulimia (3.81), GAD (3.49), separation anxiety (3.10), drug abuse (2.83), conduct disorder (2.53), dysphasia (2.51), PTSD (2.30), alcohol abuse (2.27), major depression (2.18) and social phobia (2.0) (Plana-Ripoll et al. 2019).

10. Medical Comorbidities: Schizophrenia, mood disorders and anxiety disorders are all associated with a significant increase in various medical illnesses (Momen et al. 2020). In gene-wide association studies (GWAS) of schizophrenia, the histo-compatibility complex genetic locus on chromosome 6 was significantly abnormal compared to healthy controls. This points to immune dysregulation that may predispose to many physical diseases of the body and the brain.

11. The 'P' factor: Multiple reports have suggested the presence of a single shared psychopathological predisposition to various dimensions of psychiatric disorders called the 'P' factor (Caspi and Moffitt 2018; Caspi et al. 2014; Nasrallah 2015; Selzami et al. 2018). Kendler (2019) elaborated on the conceptual evolution within psychiatric nosology from one disorder prior to the introduction of the DSM, to numerous disorders in the DSM schema, and now back again to a single psychopathological foundation, with the accelerating evidence for a unified model that stands in contrast to the widely held current DSM model.

In conclusion, it is quite evident that transformative changes may be forth coming in the diagnostic framework of psychiatric disorders. That will represent a seismic change to the DSM structure as it currently exists. This book is an important compilation of the emerging evidence for a transdiagnostic model of mental illness generated from the shared genes, environmental factors, brain circuits and neurobiological processes. The authors are to be thanked and commended for assembling an excellent volume that may serve as a catalyst for the urgently needed disruptive transformation in re-conceptualizing the transdiagnostic underpinnings of psychiatric disorders. Once adopted, the new model may lead to therapeutic innovations and brave new treatment modalities and interventions that can exploit the many overlapping comorbidities of the schizophrenia syndrome.

Henry A. Nasrallah, MD
University of Cincinnati
College of Medicine

REFERENCES

Beauchaine TP, Constantino JN (2017) Redefining the endophenotype concept to accommodate transdiagnostic vulnerabilities and etiological complexity. Biomarkers in Medicine 11: 769–780.

Beauchaine TP, Constantino JN, Hayden EP (2018) Psychiatry and developmental psychopathology: unifying themes and future directions. Comprehensive Psychiatry 87: 143–152.

Caspi A, Houts RM, Belsky DW, et al. (2014) The P factor: one general psychopathology factor in the structure of psychiatric disorders? Clinical Psychological Science 2: 119–137.

Caspi A, Moffitt TE (2018) All for one and one for all; mental disorders in one dimension. American Journal of Psychiatry 175: 831–844.

Doernberg E, Hollender E (2016) Neurodevelopmental disorders (ASD and ADHD): DSM-5, ICD-10, and ICD-11. CNS Spectrums 21: 295–299.

Elliott ML, Romer A, Knodt AR, et al. (2018) A connectome-wide functional signature of transdiagnostic risk for mental illness. Biological Psychiatry 84: 452–459.

Etkin A, Cuthbert B (2014) Beyond the DSM: development of a transdiagnostic psychiatric neuroscience course. Academic Psychiatry 38: 145–150.

Goodkind M, Eickoff SB, Oathes DJ, et al. (2015) Identification of a common neurobiological substrate for mental illness. JAMA Psychiatry 72: 305–315.

Grisanzio KA, Goldstein-Piekarski AN, Wang MY, et al. (2018) Transdiagnostic symptom clusters and associations with brain behavior and daily function in mood anxiety and trauma disorders. JAMA Psychiatry 75: 201–209.

Gudmundsson DO, Walters GB, Ingason A, et al. (2019) Attention-deficit hyperactivity disorder shares copy number variant risk with schizophrenia and autism spectrum disorder. Translational Psychiatry 9: 258. doi: 10.1038/s41398-019-0599-y.

Huttunen MO, Mednick SA (2018) Polyvagal theory, neurodevelopment and psychiatric disorders. Indian Journal of Psychological Medicine 35: 9–10.

Hyman S (2019) New evidence for shared risk architecture of mental disorders. JAMA Psychiatry 76: 235–236.

Kendler KS (2019) From many to one to many—the search for causes of psychiatric illness. JAMA Psychiatry (2019) 76: 1085–1091.

Kessler RC, Ormel J, Petukhora M, et al. (2011) Development of life-time comorbidity in the World Health Organization world mental health surveys. Archives of General Psychiatry 68: 90–100.

Krueger RF, Eaton NR (2015) Transdiagnostic factors of mental disorders. World Psychiatry 14: 27–29.

Maher AR, Theodore G (2012) Summary of the comparative review on off-label use of atypical antipsychotics. Journal of Managed Care & Specialty Pharmacy (Suppl.) 18: S1–S20.

Marshal M (2020) Roots of mental illness, researchers are beginning to untangle the common biology that links supposedly distinct psychiatric conditions. Nature 581: 19–21.

Momen NC, Plana-Ripollo O, Agerbo E, et al. (2020) Association between mental disorders and subsequent medical conditions. New England Journal of Medicine 382: 1721–1731.

Nasrallah HA (2017) Beyond DSM-5: clinical and biologic features shared by major psychiatric syndromes. Current Psychiatry 16: 4–7.

Nasrallah HA (2015) Is there only 1 neurological disorder, with different clinical expression? Current Psychiatry 14: 10–12.

Nasrallah HA (2013) Pleiotropy of psychiatric disorders will re-invent DSM. Current Psychiatry 12: 6–7.

Nasrallah HA (2019) Psychosis as a common thread across psychiatric disorders. Current Psychiatry 18: 12–14.

Plana-Ripoll O, Pedersen CB, Holtz Y, et al. (2019) Exploring comorbidity within mental disorders among a Danish national population. JAMA Psychiatry 76: 259–270.

Selzami S, Coleman JRI, Caspi A, et al. (2018) A polygenic P factor for major psychiatric disorder. Translational Psychiatry 8: 205 (pages 1–9).

Smoller J and the Cross-Disorder Group of the Psychiatric Genomics Consortium (2019) Genomic relationships, novel loci, and pleiotropic mechanisms across eight psychiatric disorders. Cell 179: 1469–1482.

Xia CH, Ma Z, Ciric R, et al. (2018) Linked dimensions of psychopathology and connectivity in functional brain networks. Nature Communications 9: 1–14.

Preface

Psychiatric comorbidities such as depression, anxiety and substance use are extremely common amongst people with schizophrenia. They add to poor clinical outcomes and disability yet are often not at the forefront of the minds of clinicians, who tend to concentrate on assessing and treating the core symptoms of schizophrenia, notably delusions and hallucinations. There is an imperative to assess every patient with schizophrenia for psychiatric comorbidities, as they might masquerade as core psychotic symptoms (e.g. depression presenting as negative symptoms) and also because they warrant treatment in their own right.

There are other psychiatric comorbidities associated with schizophrenia that tease at the very nosological constructs upon which modern psychiatry is based. These include personality disorders and neurodevelopmental disorders such as attention deficit disorder and autism spectrum disorder.

This volume addresses these issues using a clinical lens informed by the current literature. We cover nosology, epidemiology and aetiology, but our main foci are clinical aspects such as assessment and treatment. Clinical pointers, summary fact boxes, summary tables and illustrations are used to make the book appealing and reader-friendly.

This volume represents the third in a series under the *Oxford Psychiatry Library* marque: companion volumes are *Schizophrenia*, now in its second edition (Castle and Buckley 2015) which was highly commended by the British Medical Association (2015), and *Physical Health and Schizophrenia* (Castle, Buckley, and Gaughran 2017). We believe that this current book augments these previous works and will be of interest to all those involved in the care of people with schizophrenia.

We are most grateful to Oxford University Press for their support in the production of this book and trust we have succeeded in our aims of highlighting the importance of understanding, assessing and treating effectively psychiatric comorbidities in schizophrenia.

David J. Castle, Peter F. Buckley, and Rachel Upthegrove
May 2020

Contents

Abbreviations

ALSPAC	Avon Longitudinal Study of Parents and Children
ASD	autism spectrum disorder
BAP	British Association for Psychopharmacology
BPD	borderline personality disorder
BSNIP	Bipolar Schizophrenia Network on Intermediate Phenotypes
CBD	cannabidiol
CBT	cognitive behavioural therapy
CBTp	cognitive behavioural therapy for psychosis
CDS	Calgary Depression Scale
CNV	copy number variants
DMN	default mode network
DSM-5	Diagnostic and Statistical Manual of Mental Diseases, Fifth Edition
EAGLES	Evaluating Adverse Events in a Global Smoking Cessation Study
ECA	epidemiological catchment area
ECT	electroconvulsive therapy
EMDR	eye movement desensitization and reprocessing
EPSE	extrapyramidal side effects
FEP	first episode psychosis
FGA	first generation agents
GAD	generalized anxiety disorder
GWAS	genome-wide association study
KF	Kayser Fleischer
LAI	long-acting injectable antipsychotics
LSAS	Liebowitz Social Anxiety Scale
MI	motivational interviewing
NICE	National Institute for Health and Care Excellence
NPSAE	neuropsychiatric adverse event
NRT	nicotine replacement therapies
OCD	obsessive compulsive disorder
OCS	obsessive compulsive symptoms
OR	odds ratio
PD	panic disorder
PGC	Psychiatric Genomics Consortium
PPD	paranoid personality disorder
PRS	polygenic risk score

PTSD	post-traumatic stress disorder
QTc	corrected QT interval
RDC	research domain criteria
RIMA	reversible inhibitors of monoamine oxidase A
rsFC	resting state functional connectivity
SGA	second generation antipsychotic
SHIP	Survey of High Impact Psychoses
SMD	standardized mean difference
SNRI	serotonin noradrenaline reuptake inhibitor
SPD	schizotypal personality disorder
SRI	serotonergic reuptake inhibitor
SSD	schizophrenia spectrum disorder
SSRI	selective serotonin reuptake inhibitor
TF-CBT	trauma focused cognitive behavioural therapy
TTFC	time to first cigarette
UHR	ultra-high risk

CHAPTER 1

Psychiatric comorbidities associated with schizophrenia: how should we conceptualize them?

> **KEY POINTS**
>
> * Schizophrenia carries a high rate of psychiatric comorbidities.
> * Such comorbidities worsen the longitudinal course of illness and perturb treatments.
> * Genetic studies point to substantial overlap in genes across many psychiatric disorders, with no 'purity' for specific disorders.
> * Understanding the neurobiology of symptom sets might enhance models explaining overlapping symptoms between and across psychiatric disorders.

That other psychiatric conditions occur with high frequency among people with schizophrenia is—as evidenced throughout this book—both compelling and ir-refutable. Differing sampling methods, heterogeneity among schizophrenia samples studied, and cross sectional or longitudinal study designs do not obscure or detract from the repetitive finding of high rates of psychiatric comorbidities in schizophrenia (Buckley et al. 2009; Hwang and Buckley 2018; Miller et al. 2009; Yum et al. 2016). Medical conditions are also overrepresented in people with schizophrenia (Meyer and Nasrallah 2009). Rates of occurrences of psychiatric comorbidities can certainly be debated, though they are in the order of preva-lence rates of 50% for depression in schizophrenia, 47% for substance abuse, 29% for post-traumatic stress disorder (PTSD), 23% for obsessive compulsive dis-order (OCD), and 15% for panic disorder (Miller et al. 2009). Taken collectively, it is highly likely that a clinician treating a person with schizophrenia over several years will be faced with managing one or more of these psychiatric comorbidities. That said, we know that such comorbidities are associated with poorer outcomes (Gregory et al. 2017) and with more complicated pharmacotherapy; the choices therein also contribute to more adverse side effects. Thus, at its most funda-mental, psychiatric comorbidities are important in schizophrenia because they occur 'more than chance'; they are common in the aggregate; they complicate treatment; and they confer a poorer course of schizophrenia illness (Box 1.1).

Box 1.1 Putative rationale for the heightened association between schizophrenia and other psychiatric conditions

- More than chance occurrence
- Diagnostic overlap and confusion about phenomenology
- 'Blurred boundaries' of schizophrenia
- Shared neurobiology—genetic and non-genetic
- Shared environmental risk factors

Hence the rationale for this dedicated book, wherein successive chapters detail specific associations and management strategies.

This introductory chapter aims to conceptualize these co-occurrences, to help understand the overall context as well as any nuances related to specific comorbidities, and thereupon to 'set the stage' for successive chapters, especially the upcoming chapter that details the prevalence and diagnostic conundrum associated with these comorbidities.

The boundaries of schizophrenia are blurred

The most compelling, and indeed intriguing, context begins with schizophrenia itself. The notion of additional psychiatric conditions that are at the very least some way symptomatically different from schizophrenia builds upon the assumption that schizophrenia is itself a distinct, recognizable and circumscribed condition (Fischer and Carpenter 2009; McCutcheon et al. 2020). Ideally, of course, this 'illness' would then be further defined by a distinct neurobiological architecture. Notwithstanding the seminal work of Kraepelin (1912) in clinically delineating schizophrenia ('dementia praecox') from bipolar disorder ('manic-depressive insanity'), the demarcation of the nosology and consequent diagnostic boundaries of schizophrenia is anything but sharp and distinct. Schizophrenia is actually notoriously heterogeneous in its clinical aspects—in onset and presentation, in symptoms, in course over time, and ultimately in treatment and prognosis (McCutcheon et al. 2020). Even while the conceptual model of schizophrenia is still debated, there exists evidence of underlying neurobiological heterogeneity as well as a contrast to other conditions. In medicine, consider the uncommon condition of Wilson's disease, which is readily and reliably diagnosed when copper-deposited rings—Kayser Fleischer (KF) rings—are seen on slip lamp ophthalmological evaluation. KF rings are pathognomonic of Wilson's disease. Sadly, there is presently no 'KF equivalent' for schizophrenia. This basic conceptual and nosological quandary is poignant as we now turn our attention to considering psychiatric comorbidities whose basic symptoms can, and often do, overlap with psychiatric symptoms that are usually part of the diagnosis of schizophrenia (Box 1.2).

Box 1.2 Auditory hallucinations are common in schizophrenia—though they are also observed in many other conditions

- Normal individuals
- Bipolar disorder (~ 6%)
- Unipolar, major depression (~ 20%)
- Drug abuse
- Neurological conditions—stroke, Parkinson's disease, brain tumors, cerebral trauma
- Other 'organic' psychoses (e.g. cerebral sarcoidosis)

For example, some 46% of acutely manic patients experience auditory hallucinations. Hallucinations and delusions are observed in approximately 20% of patients with major depressive disorder. Obsessions, often hard to distinguish phenomenologically from delusions, occur in about 23% of schizophrenia patients (Hwang et al. 2018). Indeed, it can be difficult to distinguish between secondary negative symptoms, depressive symptoms and primary negative symptoms. To that end, several studies comparing symptoms and even illness course across patients with schizophrenia and patients with mood disorders find more similarities than differences (Lindenmayer 2018). Additionally, drug abuse can present with a plethora of symptoms mimicking schizophrenia. Moreover, there is ample evidence that a small proportion—perhaps some 9%—of otherwise healthy individuals experience auditory hallucinations that are, albeit more attenuated, similar to those observed in patients with schizophrenia.

Does symptom overlap reflect underlying neurobiological convergence? Toward a transdiagnostic reconceptualization

Kenneth Kendler, the pre-eminent US psychiatric geneticist, once quipped 'good genes require good phenotypes' (Kendler and Diehl 1993). By that he was referring to the need to minimize clinical heterogeneity in order to study and arrive at a purer phenocopy of schizophrenia. Yet, even in his meticulously conducted Roscommon studies of schizophrenia wherein the diagnosis of schizophrenia in the proband was assigned with great rigor, Kendler observed that the genetics of schizophrenia were not 'pure' (Kendler and Gardner 1997). That is to say, in addition to heightened rates of schizophrenia (compared with the general population) in primary relatives, the family members also had higher rates of schizotypal personality disorder, of bipolar disorder, of major depression, and of paranoid personality disorder. These are well-replicated findings (Glahn et al. 2014). Fast forward to the present era of ever more sophisticated genetics and large sample sizes and one observes that the overlap in genetic architecture is now more apparent among schizophrenia and several other psychiatric disorders. In a seminal paper reporting on some 100,000 persons in a genome-wide association study (GWAS) (Schizophrenia Working Group of the Psychiatric Genomics Consortium 2014), the Psychiatric Genomics Consortium (PGC) identified 108 loci associated with schizophrenia with broad implications for pathophysiology—especially with overlap with the immune system. Another paper by Gandal and colleagues (2018) detailed the genetic and transcription overlap across postmortem brains from patients with schizophrenia, bipolar disorder, depression, autism, or alcoholism in comparison with the brains of normal subjects. In contrast to expectations, these researchers observed considerable overlap across each psychiatric condition—surprisingly with alcoholism being the most divergent—and strong overlap between schizophrenia and mood disorders, both bipolar disorder and (lesser so) depression and also between schizophrenia and autism. They postulated an overall similarity of neurobiology giving way to divergence of neuropathology at a molecular level. In another GWAS (Cross-Disorder Group of the Psychiatric Genomics Consortium 2013) of around 33,000 patients with major psychiatric disorders, there was overlap between schizophrenia, bipolar disorder, major depression, autism and attention deficit disorder, particularly implicating genes in calcium signalling. Andlauer and colleagues (2019) examined 395 individuals from multiple bipolar disorder families and observed higher polygenic risk scores for both bipolar disorder and schizophrenia. And Pasman et al. (2018) showed overlap in genes predisposing to both schizophrenia and cannabis use. Taken together, these modern-day genetic analyses suggest some shared genetic vulnerability and marked transdiagnostic heritability for major psychiatric conditions (Box 1.3).

Other neurobiological studies across schizophrenia and mood disorders point to a similar convergence of neurobiological findings. Tamminga and colleagues (Pearlson et al. 2016; Tamminga et al. 2014) examined the Bipolar Schizophrenia Network on Intermediate Phenotypes (BSNIP) database and found no meaningful differences across neuroimaging and electroencephalogram (EEG) parameters among patients with schizophrenia, schizoaffective disorder and bipolar disorder. In contrast, they reported three 'intermediate phenotypes' that they call 'biotypes'. These biotypes reflect three distinct consistent patterns of neurobiological abnormalities that do not map coherently onto the expression of schizophrenia,

---

Box 1.3 A transdiagnostic perspective on major mental illness: conditions that show greater (than otherwise expected) genetic convergence

- Schizophrenia
- Bipolar disorder
- Unipolar depression
- Autism
- Attention deficit disorder

schizoaffective disorder, or bipolar disorder. This constellation, they hypothesize, reflects some neurobiological signature(s) of psychoses. De Zwarte and colleagues (2019), reporting for the ENIGMA neuroimaging study, found similar neuroimaging findings in relatives of first-episode schizophrenia patients and in relatives of probands with bipolar disorder. Another position emission tomography study (Jauhar et al. 2017) found essentially similar dopamine receptor sensitivity across schizophrenia and bipolar disorder. Moser and colleagues (2018) conducted an magnetic resonance imaging (MRI) study of 100 patients with schizophrenia and 40 patients with bipolar disorder compared with normal volunteers. They described patterns of cortical dysconnectivity and volume changes that correlated better with symptoms than with diagnosis. This is suggestive of more distinct neuroimaging phenotypes than the more traditional clinical diagnoses.

Unifying themes and nuanced observations on discrete psychiatric comorbidities

The convergence of recent genetic findings across schizophrenia and other major psychiatric conditions is both intriguing and puzzling (Box 1.4). The findings may point to shared genetic liability that is manifest in life in different symptom constellations because of other selective genetic risks, environmental risks, or any combination of both (Glahn et al. 2014; Muller 2017; Radua et al. 2018). Additionally, this genetic overlap may be related to fundamental pathogenic processes that might be in play, more or less, for a given psychiatric condition. For example, the 108 loci observed in the seminal paper by PGC in *Nature* (2014) found that these loci were also associated with immune functions. There is robust literature on immune dysfunction in mood disorders and similar findings are now evident for schizophrenia (Muller 2017). Also, developmental genes have been implicated in the GWAS of schizophrenia and major psychiatric disorders, perhaps implicating an underlying and shared neurodevelopmental basis to several psychiatric conditions in addition to schizophrenia (de Zwarte et al. 2019).

This blurring of neurobiological boundaries, coupled with the fluctuating nature of psychotic symptoms, has led to a reconsideration of more broad transdiagnostic approaches in trying to understanding and classify psychiatric conditions (Fusar-Poli et al. 2019). In that context, then, the distinctions between

---

Box 1.4 Putative neurobiological mechanisms to explain the heightened association between schizophrenia and other psychiatric conditions

- Shared genes implicating a fundamental dysregulation of the immune system
- Shared genes implicating shared neurodevelopmental basics
- Shared non-genetic risk factors (e.g. obstetric complications, 'season of birth' effect, implicating neurodevelopmental processes)

what is 'schizophrenia' and what is an 'additional' psychiatric comorbidity seem less distinct and rigorous. Moreover, this approach lines up well with the high prevalence of comorbidities in schizophrenia.

It is also noteworthy, observing through the pharmacologic lens, that medication effects of major psychiatric drugs may not be as disease-specific or even symptom-targeted as one might expect from their development. Indeed, many of the second-generation antipsychotic medications (SGAs) have demonstrated unequivocal efficiency in mood disorders and even in 'non-psychotic' major depression (Gregory et al. 2018; Goff 2019). Conversely, antidepressant medications have been shown to improve negative symptoms in schizophrenia and not (merely) treat comorbid depressive symptoms. For example, Goff and colleagues (2019) reported on a one-year, double-blind, placebo-controlled trial of citalopram in patients with first episode of psychosis. Citalopram was found to have a modest effect on negative symptoms, while depressive symptoms were similar between citalopram-treated and placebo-treated patients. Also, intriguingly, clozapine has been robustly observed to have an antisuicide effect in patients with schizophrenia (Meltzer et al. 2003).

Some concluding observations are relevant to selective psychiatric comorbidities. In addiction disorders, some drugs (e.g. cannabis, amphetmaines, ketamine) show high propensity to induce psychosis and to 'bring on' schizophrenia, while other drugs (e.g. heroin, inhalants) do not appear to have such an effect (Arendt et al. 2008; Clerici et al. 2018; Starzer et al. 2018; Voce et al. 2018). It is suggested that the heightened risk for schizophrenia among cannabis abusers reflects (hyper-)dopaminergic dysregulation. Similarly, for ketamine-related psychoses it is suggested that glutamate receptor antagonism causes a hyper-glutamatergic state that is responsible for this psychosis. In depression comorbidity, leaving aside the potential for shared genetic and environmental liabilities, there is the very real potential that people who experience psychosis may have 'insight-related' depression and grieving experiences.

In conclusion, this chapter presents a genetic and neurobiological lens to help elucidate our conceptualization(s) for the frequent clinical overlap between schizophrenia and other psychiatric conditions. Subsequent chapters 'drill down' into these associations, address psychosocial aspects of the comorbidity between schizophrenia and other psychiatric disorders, and provide an overview of clinical management thereupon.

REFERENCES

Andlauer TRM, Guzman-Parra J, Streit F, et al. (2019) Bipolar multiplex families have an increased burden of common risk variants for psychiatric disorders. Molecular Psychiatry Nov 11, doi: 10.1038/s41380-019-0558-2.

Arendt M, Mortensen PB, Rosenberg R, et al. (2008) Familial predisposition for psychiatric disorder: comparison of subjects treated for cannabis-induced psychosis and schizophrenia. Archives of General Psychiatry 65: 1269–1274.

Buckley PF, Miller BJ, Lehrer DS, Castle DJ (2009) Psychiatric comorbidities and schizophrenia. Schizophrenia Bulletin 35: 383–402.

Clerici M, de Bartolomeis A, De Filippis S, et al. (2018) Patterns of management of patients with dual disorder (psychosis) in Italy: a survey of psychiatrists and other physicians focusing on clinical practice. Frontiers in Psychiatry 9: 575.

Cross-Disorder Group of the Psychiatric Genomics Consortium (2013) Identification of risk loci with shared effects on five major psychiatric disorders: a genome-wide analysis. Lancet, doi: 10.1016/S0140-6739(12)62129-1.

de Zwarte SMC, Brouwer RM, Agartz I, et al. (2019) The association between familial risk and brain abnormalities is disease specific: an ENIGMA-relatives study of schizophrenia and bipolar disorder. Biological Psychiatry 86: 545–556.

Fischer BA, Carpenter WT Jr (2009) Will the Kraepelinian dichotomy survive DSM-V? Neuropsychopharmacology 34: 2081–2087.

Fusar-Poli P, Solmi M, Brondino N, et al. (2019) Transdiagnostic psychiatry: a systematic review. World Psychiatry 18: 192–207.

Gandal MJ, Haney JR, Parikshak NN, et al. (2018) Shared molecular neuropathology across major psychiatric disorders parallels polygenic overlap. Science 359: 693–697.

Glahn DC, Knowles EE, McKay DR, et al. (2014) Arguments for the sake of endophenotypes: examining common misconceptions about the use of endophenotypes in psychiatric genetics. American Journal of Medical Genetics B: Neuropsychiatric Genetics 165: 122–130.

Goff DC, Freudenreich O, Cather C, et al. (2019) Citalopram in first episode schizophrenia: the DECIFER trial. Schizophrenia Research 208: 331–337.

Gregory A, Mallikarjun P, Upthegrove R (2017) Treatment of depression in schizophrenia: systematic review and meta-analysis. British Journal of Psychiatry 211: 198–204.

Hwang M, Buckley P (2018) Comorbidity and schizophrenia. Psychiatric Annals 48: 544–545.

Hwang M, Sood A, Riaz B, Poyurovsky M (2018) Obsessive-compulsive schizophrenia: clinical and conceptual perspective. Psychiatric Annals 48: 552–556.

Jauhar S, Nour MM, Veronese M, et al. (2017) A test of the transdiagnostic dopamine hypothesis of psychosis using positron emission tomographic imaging in bipolar affective disorder and schizophrenia. JAMA Psychiatry 74: 1206–1213.

Kendler KS, Diehl SR (1993) The genetics of schizophrenia: a current, genetic-epidemiologic perspective. Schizophrenia Bulletin 19: 261–285.

Kendler, KS, Gardner CO (1997) The risk for psychiatric disorders in relatives of schizophrenic and control probands: a comparison of three independent studies. Psychological Medicine 27: 411–419.

Kraepelin E (1912) Psychiatry: a textbook for students and physicians, 7th edition. Leipzig: MacMillan.

Lindenmayer JP (2018) The NIMH research domain criteria initiative and comorbidity in schizophrenia: research implications. Psychiatric Annals 48: 547–551.

McCutcheon RA, Marques TR, Howes OD (2020) Schizophrenia—an overview. JAMA Psychiatry 77: 201–210.

Meltzer HY, Alphs L, Green AI, et al. (2003) Clozapine treatment for suicidality in schizophrenia: international suicide prevention trial. Archives of General Psychiatry 60: 82–91.

Meyer JM, Nasrallah HA (2009) Medical illness and schizophrenia, 2nd edition. Washington, DC: American Psychiatric Press.

Moser DA, Doucet GE, Lee WH, et al. (2018) Multivariate associations among behavioral, clinical, and multimodal imaging phenotypes in patients with psychosis. JAMA Psychiatry 75: 386–395.

Muller N (2017) Immunological aspects of the treatment of depression and schizophrenia. Dialogues in Clinical Neuroscience 19: 55–63.

Pasman JA, Verweij KJH, Gerring Z, et al. (2018) GWAS of lifetime cannabis use reveals new risk loci, genetic overlap with psychiatric traits and a causal influence of schizophrenia. Nature Neuroscience 21: 1161–1170.

Pearlson GD, Clementz BA, Sweeney JA, et al. (2016) Does biology transcend the symptom-based boundaries of psychosis? Psychiatric Clinics of North America 39: 165–174.

Radua J, Ramella-Cravaro V, Loannidis JPA, et al. (2018) What causes psychosis? An umbrella review of risk and protective factors. World Psychiatry 17: 49–66.

Schizophrenia Working Group of the Psychiatric Genomics Consortium (2014) Biological insights from 108 schizophrenia associated genetic loci. Nature 65: 421–427.

Starzer MSK, Nordentoft M, Hjorthoj C (2018) Rates and predictors of conversion to schizophrenia or bipolar disorder following substance-induced psychosis. American Journal of Psychiatry 175: 343–350.

Tamminga CA, Pearlson G, Keshavan M, et al. (2014) Bipolar and schizophrenia network for intermediate phenotypes: outcomes across the psychosis continuum. Schizophrenia Bulletin 40(Suppl 2): S131–S137.

Voce A, McKetin R, Burn R, Castle D, Calabria B (2018) The relationship between illicit amphetamine use and psychiatric symptom profiles in schizophrenia and affective psychoses. Psychiatry Research 265: 19–24.

Yum, SY, Hwang, MY, Nasrallah, HA, Opler, LA (2016) Transcending psychosis—the complexity of comorbidity in schizophrenia. Psychiatric Clinics of North America 39: 267–274.

CHAPTER 2

Psychiatric comorbidities in schizophrenia: the size of the problem

KEY POINTS

- There are numerous methodological considerations to bear in mind in interpreting rates of psychiatric comorbidities in schizophrenia.
- Criterion sets used to make comorbid diagnoses vary widely and many have not been validated in people with schizophrenia.
- The sampling frame (e.g. general population vs. treated sample) as well as illness stage can impact rates of comorbidities.

This is a book about psychiatric comorbidities in schizophrenia. There are significant conceptual issues relating to the essence of what one considers 'comorbid' and how one classifies, assesses, and enumerates putative comorbid conditions. These puzzles are addressed in other chapters of this book, notably Chapters 1 and 3. In this chapter we sidestep most of those considerations and accept the conventional use of the term 'comorbid', namely another psychiatric condition occurring in a person with schizophrenia and not directly explicable as part of the manifestations of the schizophrenia itself. The established diagnostic criteria for the comorbid diagnosis need to be met, with the accepted exclusions of symptoms due to an organic process (although this is complex when it comes to substance use disorders, as detailed in Chapter 11). This allows a review of the pertinent literature regarding how often such conditions occur in people with schizophrenia as opposed to people without schizophrenia. We follow the convention that schizophrenia hierarchically 'trumps' other psychiatric disorders (see Chapter 3).

General considerations

Overall rates of psychiatric comorbidities in people with schizophrenia are dependent upon a number of methodological issues, summarized in Box 2.1. The sampling frame (i.e. general population vs. a treated population) is critical, as treated samples introduce biases related to severity of illness as well as Berkson's

---

Box 2.1 Methodological issues relevant to ascertaining rates of comorbidity in schizophrenia

- Setting (e.g. general population vs. a treatment setting)
- Ascertainment bias
- Berkson's bias
- Diagnostic criteria applied (for schizophrenia as well as for the comorbid problem under consideration)
- Skill and experience of interviewers
- Age and gender of sample
- Stage of illness
- Ethnicity
- Reporting bias (e.g. illicit drugs)
- Pathways and barriers to care for each condition
- Antipsychotic side effects

---

bias, namely the bias related to ascertainment of two or more disease entities through pathways relevant to each, thus overenumerating their co-aggregation.

Another critical issue is the diagnostic criteria applied: this is relevant to both schizophrenia and the comorbid condition. Schizophrenia itself has undergone many alterations in its definition over the last century. A full exposition of these changes is beyond the scope of this book and the reader is referred to the companion book in this series for details (Castle and Buckley 2015). A summary is provided in Box 2.2. Perhaps of most importance to this chapter are the

---

Box 2.2 Selected overview of changes in the schizophrenia construct, over time, relevant to psychiatric comorbidities

- Kraepelin (1896): early onset, male preponderant 'neurodevelopmental'-type illness
- Bleuler (1911): broader criteria and notion of 'group of schizophrenias'; differentiation of primary and secondary criterion sets
- Feighner (1974): restrictive criteria loading towards early onset (under age 40 years) and family history of schizophrenia
- Research Domain Criteria (RDC) (1976): broader criteria
- ICD-9 (1970s): broad definition not operationalized
- DSM-III (1980): age at onset stipulated as under 45 years
- ICD-10 (1990): no age at onset stipulation
- DSM-IV (1987): abandoned age at onset stipulation
- DSM-5 (2013): moved away from emphasis on Schniederian 'first rank' symptoms; abandoned subtypes

---

variations in age at onset, as psychiatric comorbidities affect individuals at different life phases, as outlined below. Feighner criteria for schizophrenia loaded towards early onset cases (under 40 years), DSM-III specified an onset before the age of 45 years, but DSM-IV dropped any age specification. Another related issue is the impact on sex ratios of the different sets of criteria. For example, Feighner's criteria preference males, with an estimated male:female ratio of 2.5:1, whilst DSM-III returns a ratio of 2.2:1, and more 'liberal' criteria with age at onset specifications, such as ICD-9, estimate males and females to be roughly even in terms of schizophrenia risk (Castle et al. 1993). Sex affects psychiatric comorbidities in important ways, again as detailed below. Finally, quirky criteria within certain diagnostic sets will serve to prejudice against finding high rates of psychiatric comorbidities, for example the loading for a family history of schizophrenia in Feighner's criteria.

As alluded to above, the age and sex of the sample is likely to impact estimates of psychiatric comorbidities. This can be a function of the diagnostic criteria applied (see Box 2.1) and/or the sampling frame. If the schizophrenia sample is of older females, there is a likelihood of overestimating other psychiatric conditions that tend to afflict people of that demographic: depression and certain of the anxiety disorders, for example. Conversely, a sample of young males with schizophrenia will likely show higher comorbid neurodevelopmental disorders such as autism spectrum disorders.

Stage of illness is important. The onset of schizophrenia can be profoundly traumatic for the individual, related to both the symptoms of psychosis as well as treatment issues (e.g. forced hospitalization, forced medication, seclusion and restraint), whilst cumulative trauma across the illness course can be expected to impact rates of post-traumatic syndromes: these issues are addressed in detail in Chapter 9. Hall (2017) has emphasized the high rates of generalized anxiety symptoms in the schizophrenia prodrome, as well as in the phases preceding relapse. Similarly, high rates of depression have been recorded in first episode patients (see Chapter 10). Conversely, OCD becomes more commonly comorbid with schizophrenia as the illness progresses: thus, in a recent-onset cohort of schizophrenia patients, rates of OCD would be lower than if people are ascertained later on in their illness course (see Chapter 8).

Culture and ethnicity can introduce bias. For example, some ethnic groups may be more likely to use certain substances, whilst help-seeking and/or expression of the anxiety disorders might be impacted by cultural and ethnic parameters. Jurisdictional issues pertain as legal attitudes to drugs such as cannabis can impact availability and general population rates of use: reporting bias might operate, with people being potentially less likely to divulge the use of substances if they are illegal.

The importance of the antipsychotic medication prescribed to the individual being assessed for psychiatric comorbidities lies largely in the side effect burden of individual agents, as these might induce, exacerbate, or masquerade as psychiatric disorders. Examples of the former include the induction or exacerbation of obsessive compulsive symptoms by many of the atypical antipsychotics, notably clozapine (see Chapter 8); and likewise for depressive symptoms with some of the typical agents (see Chapter 10). Antipsychotic-induced extrapyramidal side effects, notably restriction of affect and avolition, may masquerade as depression, whilst akathisia can be misinterpreted as anxiety.

Rate estimates

Given all these issues, it is hardly surprising that there is a great deal of variation in estimates of psychiatric comorbidities in schizophrenia. Other chapters of this book interrogate these rates for specific disorders. Here we provide overall estimates. Where recent systematic reviews and summary rate estimates are available, these are given.

There are particular difficulties ascertaining rates of other neurodevelopmental disorders in people with schizophrenia, in part due to overlap of symptoms and problems determining primacy. The systematic review of De Giorgi and colleagues (2019) returned a weighted average prevalence rate of psychosis of 9.5% among people with autism spectrum disorders.

The same problems pertain to the personality disorders, notably those in which core features are shared with schizophrenia itself: this is the case for schizoid, schizotypal, and paranoid personality disorders, and people with borderline personality disorder can experience psychotic symptoms that are cross-sectionally difficult to distinguish from an acute exacerbation of schizophrenia. These issues are discussed in Chapter 5.

Table 2.1 tabulates findings from the meta-analysis by Achim and colleagues (2011) across numerous studies regarding anxiety disorder comorbidity in people with schizophrenia. Most of the anxiety disorders aggregate around the 10% rate (somewhat lower for agoraphobia); for 'any anxiety disorder' the rate is around 40%. This broadly concurs with the earlier review by Pokos and Castle (2006), which suggested a summary rate of around 50%, with a range from 35% to 85%.

Regarding depression, Buckley et al. (2009) reviewed 36 studies encompassing 4,447 people with schizophrenia at various stages of illness. They found a range of rates of clinically relevant depression from 5% to 65%, and concluded a mean rate could be estimated at 25%, akin to the modal rate reported by Siris and Bench (2003). In Chapter 10, a cross-sectional rate of 25–30% is quoted, with acknowledgement that higher rates (around 50%) are found in longitudinal studies and even higher rates (up to 80%) in first episode patients.

Rates of substance use and abuse amongst people with schizophrenia likewise vary greatly across samples, reflecting different methods of ascertainment, different phases of illness, and jurisdictional issues, as outlined above. Chapter 11 deals with these issues in detail, but a 'take home' overall prevalence rate for illicit substance use amongst people with schizophrenia of 40–60%, is defensible (Cantor-Graae et al. 2001).

Table 2.1 Prevalence rates of anxiety disorders comorbid with schizophrenia

Disorder	Number of studies (n)	Number of patients (n)	Mean prevalence rate (%) (95% CI)	Range (%)
OCD	34	3007	12.1 (7.0–17.1)	0.6–55.0
Panic disorder	23	1393	9.8 (4.3–15.4)	0.0–35.0
Agoraphobia	12	862	5.4 (0.2–10.6)	0.0–27.5
PTSD	20	1388	12.4 (4.0–20.8)	0.0–51.4
Social phobia	16	1259	14.9 (8.1–21.8)	3.6–39.5
Specific phobia	11	925	7.9 (1.9–13.8)	0.0–30.8
Generalized anxiety disorder (GAD)	14	939	10.9 (2.9–18.8)	0.0–45
Any anxiety disorder	16	958	38.3 (26.3–50.4)	10.4–85.0

Adapted with permission from Achim, A. M., Maziade, M., Raymond, E., et al. How prevalent are anxiety disorders in schizophrenia? A meta-analysis and critical review of a significant association. *Schizophrenia Bulletin*, 37: 811–821. © The Author 2011. Published by Oxford University Press on behalf of the Maryland Psychiatric Research Center. All rights reserved.

Conclusions

Reported rates of psychiatric comorbidities in people with schizophrenia show marked variation across studies, dependent upon a number of methodological issues including sampling frame, diagnostic instruments employed, stage of illness, and a number of demographic variables. What is consistent across studies is that rates across all psychiatric disorders are higher amongst people with schizophrenia than in people without a mental illness. The imperative for clinicians is to be aware of the extent of such comorbidities in their patients and to ensure they screen for these maladies, as there are profound implications for treatment. These issues are discussed in more detail in the individual treatment chapters in this book.

REFERENCES

Achim AM, Maziade M, Raymond E, et al. (2011) How prevalent are anxiety disorders in schizophrenia? A meta-analysis and critical review of a significant association. Schizophrenia Bulletin 37: 811–821.

Buckley PF, Miller BJ, Lehrer DS, Castle DJ (2009) Psychiatric comorbidities and schizophrenia. Schizophrenia Bulletin 35: 383–402.

Cantor-Graae E, Nordstrom LG, McNeil TF (2001) Substance abuse in schizophrenia: a review of the literature and a study of correlates in Sweden. Schizophrenia Research 48: 69–82.

Castle DJ, Buckley PF (2015) Schizophrenia. Oxford: Oxford University Press.

Castle DJ, Wessely S, Murray RM (1993) Sex and schizophrenia: effects of diagnostic stringency, and associations with premorbid variables. British Journal of Psychiatry 162: 658–664.

De Giorgi R, De Crescenzo F, D'Alo G, et al. (2019) Prevalence of non-affective psychoses in individuals with autism spectrum disorders: a systematic review. Journal of Clinical Medicine 8: 1304.

Hall J (2017) Schizophrenia: an anxiety disorder? British Journal of Psychiatry 211: 262–263.

Pokos V, Castle DJ (2006) Prevalence of comorbid anxiety disorders in schizophrenia spectrum disorders: a literature review. Current Psychiatry Reviews 2: 285–307.

Siris S, Bench C (2003) Depression and schizophrenia. In: Hirsch S, Weinberger D (eds) Schizophrenia, 2nd edition. Oxford: Blackwell, pp. 142–167.

CHAPTER 3

Why are psychiatric comorbidities so common in schizophrenia and why are they so often missed in clinical practice?

KEY POINTS

* The comorbidity of schizophrenia with other psychiatric disorders needs to be considered in the context of key nosological constraints.
* Numerous different pathways need to be explored in building a model of comorbidity.
* Clinicians need always to ask questions about comorbid symptoms.
* Clinicians must avoid falling into the trap of labelling all symptoms and behaviours of the individual as due to schizophrenia itself.

The extent of psychiatric comorbidities in schizophrenia is well documented in Chapter 2 of this book. An excess risk is evident across the board, from early neurodevelopmental disorders such as autism and attention deficit disorder, through depression and all the anxiety disorders, as well as post-traumatic syndromes and OCD, and also encompassing substance use disorders. This chapter seeks to understand why these disorders are so common in people with schizophrenia, and also asks why they are so commonly missed in clinical practice. Subsequent chapters deal with each disorder in turn; hence this chapter provides an overview and conceptual working model. The reader is referred specifically to Chapter 1 for an overarching framework.

Why are comorbid psychiatric disorders so common in people with schizophrenia?

Semantic and nosological issues

Broadly, we can approach this question by addressing biological, psychological, and social determinants. But we also need to consider semantic issues. In hierarchical models of mental illness (see Figure 3.1) there is a tendency—mostly pragmatic and treatment-informed—to give schizophrenia status near the top of the pyramid. Only 'organic' factors 'trump' schizophrenia. Again, this is sensible

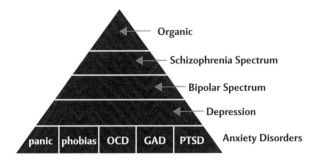

Figure 3.1 A representation of the hierarchical model of mental illness.
Adapted with permission from Castle, D., Bassett, D., King, J., Gleason, A. (eds) *A Primer of Clinical Psychiatry*, 2nd Edition, Oxford University Press: Oxford, copyright © 2013, Elsevier Australia.

in many ways but does beg questions about where 'organic' ends and 'functional' begins.

The exclusion from a diagnosis of schizophrenia of psychotic symptoms occurring in the context of a brain tumour makes perfect sense and has profound treatment implications. But an exclusion of the diagnosis in people who happen to be using a psychotomimetic drug is far more difficult to sustain. As outlined in Chapter 11, substance use and abuse are very common amongst people with schizophrenia, and some of these substances (e.g. cannabis) seem to raise the overall risk of the illness, bring forward the onset, and certainly make relapse more likely. Hence such drugs arguably act in concert with other factors, perturbing the dopamine system, acting as a cumulative causal factor, and triggering episodes of illness (Castle 2013). In such individuals a primary diagnosis of schizophrenia is applied and substance abuse is considered comorbid: as articulated in Chapter 11, we refer to this as 'drug precipitated'. But the nosological status of those individuals who have repeated psychotic episodes in response to use of stimulant drugs such as methamphetamine remains uncertain, especially when after years of such exposure they develop a syndrome that looks to all intents and purposes like 'schizophrenia' (Voce et al. 2019).

Another conundrum is so-called schizoaffective disorder. This 'nosological inconvenience', as it has been described (Castle 2012), raises many questions about boundaries between disorders and the primacy of schizophrenia, on the one hand, and the mood disorders, on the other. Chapter 10 addresses the issue of depression in schizophrenia, essentially considering it as 'comorbid'. But in some people it can be very difficult to parse schizophrenia-like and mood-like symptoms sets, and they might show risk factors (e.g. genetic) for both sets of symptoms (see Chapter 1). Again, we tend to be pragmatic about this and develop a formulation about the person that enables effective treatment across symptoms.

But what the 'truth' is about the aetiology and nosology is as yet beyond our understanding, except at a very superficial level.

A further area of consideration is the role of trauma and the overlap between PTSD and psychosis. We know that traumatic life events are all too common in people with a mental illness, and schizophrenia is no exception. How trauma impacts people with schizophrenia is the subject of much recent research, as detailed in Chapter 9. But it is also the case that traumatic life events—notably childhood abuse—are associated with psychotic-like experiences in the general population, suggesting an impact of early trauma on the vulnerability to psychosis broadly (see Chapter 9). The obverse is that people with schizophrenia are differentially prone to various life traumas by the very nature of their illness— through experiencing terrifying delusions and hallucinations, for example, as well as through the trauma that is all too often part of treatment, notably forced treatment in hospitals, with restraint, seclusion, and forced medication. Hence there are complex interactions and causal pathways that eschew any simple binary PTSD vs. schizophrenia dichotomy.

Another problem is the overlap between autism spectrum disorders and schizophrenia (Chapter 4). One of the issues here is the fact that some features of schizophrenia itself are very much akin to those seen in autism: for example, the social awkwardness and lack of 'theory of mind' (being able to appreciate the emotions of others). Indeed, Bleuler included 'autism' as one of his primary symptoms of schizophrenia, part of what is now conceptualized as the negative symptom cluster (Castle and Buckley 2015). Hence, in a person presenting with schizophrenia—especially early onset, male preponderant 'neurodevelopmental' schizophrenia—autistic features would be considered a part of the illness itself, and a separate diagnosis of an autism spectrum disorder would seem superfluous. Yet some people with schizophrenia do have a seemingly comorbid set of symptoms warranting a discrete diagnosis of autism spectrum disorder. This is discussed in detail in Chapter 4.

Finally, the relationship of certain personality disorders to schizophrenia is confusing, as outlined in Chapter 5. Schizotypal personality disorder, for example, has many clinical features of schizophrenia itself; it tends to run in families of probands with schizophrenia; and shares a number of putative biomarkers with schizophrenia (for a full discussion and references see Chapter 5). Thus one could consider this 'personality disorder' part of the schizophrenia construct: this has been embraced by ICD-11 but not by DSM-5.

Genetic factors

Leaving aside the semantic issues raised above, there are a number of aetiological threads that tie schizophrenia to other psychiatric disorders. As discussed in Chapter 1, the genetics of schizophrenia are hugely complex and much remains to be elucidated about risk genes, gene expression, and gene–environment interaction effects. One matter that is now very clear is that there is a high degree of overlap in genetic risk across psychiatric disorders. For example, in a large-scale gene-wide association study of 33,332 people with a range of mental illnesses, there were shared risk genes across schizophrenia, autism spectrum disorder, attention deficit disorder, bipolar disorder and major depressive disorder (Cross-Disorder Group of the Psychiatric Genomics Consortium 2013). Which gene constellations predispose to which particular condition is not clear. Indeed, it is likely that no single gene is 'required' for any single psychiatric disorder, but that risk genes for some disorders are pertinent in others with similar or overlapping pathogenesis. For example, certain neurodevelopmental genes that impact neuronal migration and integration in schizophrenia would do likewise in other neurodevelopmental disorders such as autism.

Some studies have looked specifically for risk genes associated with schizophrenia and ascertained whether they are also associated with commonly comorbid disorders. For example, Power and colleagues (2014) showed that there was overlap in risk genes between schizophrenia and cannabis abuse, albeit the predictive validity was low.

Another approach is to use twin study methods, where genetic and environmental aspects of risk can be (to some degree) parsed. In one of the few such studies, Argyropoulos et al. (2008) applied additive genetic plus unique environmental risk modelling in a sample of 35 non-schizophrenia co-twins from twin pairs discordant for schizophrenia, as well as 131 control twins. There were substantially elevated rates of both depression (p = 0.006) and anxiety disorders (p = 0.021) in the non-schizophrenia co-twins compared to control twins, suggesting genetic overlap.

Other biological factors

The neurodevelopmental model of schizophrenia is now well accepted (Murray et al. 1992). In essence, it proposes that an early aberration of neural development leaves the individual vulnerable to the manifestation of schizophrenia as the brain develops in later teenage and early adult years. Whilst largely genetically determined, environmental factors such as in-utero stress and malnutrition, influenza type A, and toxoplasmosis, as well as pregnancy and birth complications can act in concert with genetic risk to increase the odds of schizophrenia developing in later life. A neurodevelopmental subtype of schizophrenia has been proposed, with the features listed in Box 3.1. It is obvious that the features show substantial overlap with other neurodevelopmental disorders such as autism, suggesting shared vulnerabilities (Chapter 4). What is not so obvious is that early-onset OCD also shows many of these features, as discussed in Chapter 8. Thus neurodevelopmental perturbations might predispose to a putative schizo-obsessive disorder, with shared features of both schizophrenia and OCD.

A further factor that is relevant to some people with schizophrenia and OCD is that certain atypical antipsychotics—notably clozapine—can exacerbate existing OCD symptoms or even cause them to arise de novo. This is discussed in more detail in Chapter 8.

Box 3.1 Features of the putative neurodevelopmental subtype of schizophrenia

* Early onset (teens, early adulthood)
* Male preponderance
* Premorbid social and intellectual dysfunction
* An excess of 'soft' neurological signs
* Subtle abnormalities in ectodermal development ('minor physical anomalies')
* Structural brain abnormalities
* Left cerebral hemisphere involvement (e.g. language)

Source: Data from Murray, R.M., O'Callaghan, E., Castle, D.J., Lewis, S.W. (1992) A neurodevelopmental approach to the classification of schizophrenia. *Schizophrenia Bulletin*, 18(2): 319–332.

A final 'biological' factor for consideration is the 'setting' of the dopamine system in individuals with schizophrenia, which leaves them more likely than other people to use and abuse dopaminergic drugs, including nicotine, cannabis, and stimulants. Indeed, as detailed in Chapter 11, people with schizophrenia endorse 'alleviation of negative affect' as the main factor driving use of such drugs. It is also the case that antipsychotics—notably the older 'typical' agents—can worsen negative affect, hence potentially enhancing cravings for drugs which can ameliorate such feelings. In contrast, clozapine may reduce the drive for use of such drugs, as discussed in Chapter 11.

Psychosocial factors

A number of adverse life factors are common across most psychiatric disorders. Traumatic life events, notably early abuse, have been noted above. Thus, the experience of such abuse could be seen as a general causal factor for psychiatric disorders and serves to increase the risk of schizophrenia as well as disorders that occur comorbidly with it. The precise mechanisms for and reasons why certain individuals develop certain psychiatric maladies in the setting of early life stress are not fully understood.

The impact of schizophrenia on an individual's life, their dislocation from society, and the stigma they experience in everyday life can often leave them feeling demoralized and depressed. Box 3.2 presents some features pertinent to this discourse. Chapter 10 discusses these factors and interactions between them in more detail.

The poor physical health of so many people with schizophrenia can add to their feelings of exclusion, shame, and lack of self-worth. Obesity, for example, carries obvious stigma in and of itself, and has strong associations with depression (Thomas et al. 2010). Sleep apnoea is common in people with schizophrenia and also serves as a risk factor for depression.

Box 3.2 Psychosocial factors associated with schizophrenia which serve as risk factors for depression

- Unemployment
- Poverty
- Social isolation
- Lack of meaningful social role
- Stigma
- Substance use
- Physical health morbidities
- Low rates of exercise
- Poor diet

Finally, the strong association between schizophrenia and substance use and abuse needs to be understood not just in terms of the biological factors outlined above, but also in terms of social affiliation and peer pressure. These broader contextual parameters are detailed in Chapter 11.

Why are psychiatric comorbidities so commonly missed in clinical practice?

Despite growing recognition of the extent of psychiatric comorbidities in people with schizophrenia, clinicians often miss them (Box 3.3). An overarching reason is that clinicians tend to focus on the 'main problem' and often simply do not ask their patients with schizophrenia any questions about symptoms, beyond the positive symptoms of the illness. A second factor is that it is all too easy to fall into the trap of 'labelling' or interpreting everything about the person through the schizophrenia lens. Thus, social withdrawal and paucity of affect are interpreted as negative symptoms rather than possibly being due to depression or anxiety.

Other factors that bedevil clinical assessment of psychiatric disorders comorbid with schizophrenia include difficulties related to the differentiation of specific symptoms as consequent upon the comorbid condition vs. due to schizophrenia (e.g. negative symptoms vs. depression; delusional obsessional symptoms as part of schizophrenia vs. OCD). Furthermore, as Achim et al. (2009) point out, delineating to what extent functional impairment is due to schizophrenia as opposed to a putative comorbid disorder can be very tricky: this has implications for any diagnostic set that mandates 'functional impairment' as part of its construct. In this context, it is important to note that few diagnostic instruments for anxiety and mood disorders have been validated for use in people with schizophrenia: a notable exception is the Calgary Depression Scale (CDS), which was specifically developed for use in people with schizophrenia and has good psychometric properties (Addington et al. 1990).

Box 3.3 Reasons for clinicians failing to diagnose comorbid psychiatric disorders in people with schizophrenia

- Over-reliance on the hierarchical model of psychiatric disorders
- Labelling theory
- Difficulty in deciding when features of comorbid disorders are not better accounted for by schizophrenia itself
- Failure to elicit specific symptoms of comorbid disorders
- Failure to assess patients when acute psychotic symptoms have settled
- Lack of diagnostic instruments for comorbid psychiatric disorders, validated for use in people with schizophrenia
- Difficulty in differentiating functional impact due to the comorbid problem as opposed to schizophrenia itself

Source: Data from Cassano, G.B., Pini, S., Saettoni, M., et al. (1998) Occurrence and clinical correlates of psychiatric comorbidity in patients with psychotic disorders. *Journal of Clinical Psychiatry*, 59: 60–68; Achim, A.M., Maziade, M., Raymond, E., et al. (2009) How prevalent are anxiety disorders in schizophrenia? A meta-analysis and critical review on a significant association. *Schizophrenia Bulletin*, 37: 811–821; Buckley, P.F., Miller, B.J., Lehrer, D.S., Castle, D.J. (2009) Psychiatric comorbidities and schizophrenia. *Schizophrenia Bulletin*, 35: 383–402.

Each chapter in this book presents ways in which schizophrenia and other psychiatric disorders might be delineated. Suffice to say here that keeping an open mind and always asking the relevant clinical questions to elicit such comorbidities should be part of every assessment of people with schizophrenia. It is particularly important to ensure the assessments are repeated when positive symptoms of psychosis have been treated, as more clarity can be brought diagnostically and it is possible to differentiate primary comorbid symptoms from those that are secondary to positive symptoms of psychosis.

Conclusions

The comorbidity of schizophrenia with other psychiatric disorders needs to be considered in the context of key nosological constraints. Numerous different pathways need to be explored in building a model of comorbidity. Clinicians need always to ask questions about comorbid symptoms and avoid falling into the trap of labelling all symptoms and behaviours of the individual as due to schizophrenia itself.

REFERENCES

Achim AM, Maziade M, Raymond E, et al. (2009) How prevalent are anxiety disorders in schizophrenia? A meta-analysis and critical review on a significant association. Schizophrenia Bulletin 37: 811–821.

Addington D, Addington J, Schissel B (1990) A depression rating scale for schizophrenics. Schizophrenia Research 3: 247–251.

Buckley PF, Miller BJ, Lehrer DS, Castle DJ (2009) Psychiatric comorbidities and schizophrenia. Schizophrenia Bulletin 35: 383–402.

Cassano GB, Pini S, Saettoni M, et al. (1998) Occurrence and clinical correlates of psychiatric comorbidity in patients with psychotic disorders. Journal of Clinical Psychiatry 59: 60–68.

Castle D (2012) Schizoaffective disorder. Advances in Psychiatric Treatment 18: 32–33.

Castle D (2013) Cannabis and psychosis: what causes what? F1000 Medicine Reports, doi: 10.3410/M5-1 F1000 Med Rep 5:1.

Castle DJ, Buckley PB (2015) Schizophrenia, 2nd edition. Oxford: Oxford University Press.

Cross-Disorder Group of the Psychiatric Genomics Consortium (2013) Identification of risk loci with shared effects on five major psychiatric disorders: a genome-wide analysis. Lancet, doi: 10.1016/S0140-6739(12)62129-1.

Murray RM, O'Callaghan E, Castle DJ, Lewis SW (1992) A neurodevelopmental approach to the classification of schizophrenia. Schizophrenia Bulletin 18: 319–332.

Power RA, Verweij KJH, Zuhair M, et al. (2014) Genetic predisposition to schizophrenia associated with increased use of cannabis. Molecular Psychiatry, doi: 10.1038/mp.2014.51.

Thomas SL, Karunaratne A, Castle D, et al. (2010) 'Just Bloody Fat!' A qualitative study of body image, self esteem and coping in obese adults. International Journal of Mental Health Promotion 12: 39–49.

Voce A, McKetin R, Burns R, et al. (2019) A systematic review of the symptom profile and course of methamphetamine use and psychotic symptoms profiles associated psychosis. Substance Use and Misuse 54: 549–559.

CHAPTER 4

Autism and schizophrenia: neurodevelopmental 'playmates'?

KEY POINTS

- Historical constructions of schizophrenia encompassed autism within their core.
- Autism and schizophrenia share certain neurodevelopmental markers, but the emphasis in autism is on reduced social awareness, restricted interests and verbal delay.
- Certain neurobiological findings overlap between autism and schizophrenia, albeit the former group tends to have larger brain volumes, whilst the latter have volume reductions in key brain areas.
- The emphases of treatment between autism and schizophrenia diverge, with the use of techniques to enhance socialization, deal with impairing behaviours, and enhance language skills being more front-and-centre in autism than schizophrenia.

To the lay public, schizophrenia and autism appear 'poles apart'. In the movie *A Beautiful Mind*, actor Russell Crowe plays the mathematics genius John Nash whose delusions, hallucinations, and resultant aberrant behaviours undermine his capacity to function. This movie well describes the features and course of schizophrenia. Similarly, the movie *Rain Man* provides a 'textbook account' of autism. In this movie, Dustin Hoffman typifies the social and verbal restrictions of autism, the idiosyncratic heightened interest/focus/skill in selective area(s), and the gross motor abnormalities of autism. A recent study of the lay public opinions of various mental illnesses confirms that people are discerning about these conditions and understanding thereupon (Butlin et al. 2019). Gratifyingly, the field of autism research has dramatically expanded over the last decade and there is a much greater understanding of both biological and psychosocial aspects of autism (Bhandari et al. 2020; Lord et al. 2020). This chapter accordingly focuses selectively on aspects of overlap between autism and schizophrenia, reflecting upon contemporary perspectives on each condition (Lord et al. 2020; McCutcheon et al. 2020; Zheng et al. 2018).

Autism and schizophrenia: historical antecedents and rates of co-occurrence

It is perhaps surprising to consider that autism and schizophrenia were at one time viewed as similar conditions. Although Euger Bleuler's use of the term

Box 4.1 Diagnostic features of autism—all longstanding and not attributable to mental retardation or other causes of developmental delays

- Restricted emotional valence
- Restricted verbal and 'body language' output
- Restricted social awareness and impoverished 'social cues'
- Tendency towards intense interest and/or activities focused in a particular area

'autism' was not synonymous with the modern-day word, Bleuler considered autism (infantile, dream-like withdrawal) as a fundamental feature of schizophrenia. And when autism was first described in a case series by Leo Kanner in 1923 it was referred to as 'Kanner's psychosis'. Subsequent descriptions by other leading child psychiatrists, foremost among them the British psychiatrist Sir Michael Rutter, clarified that the features of autism were largely different from schizophrenia and that there was a reliability of presentation and course to be able to describe autism as a distinct condition. As described in the Diagnostic and Statistical Manual of Mental Diseases, Fifth Edition (DSM-5, 2013), the core features of autism are across several domains and still do show some potential for overlap with schizophrenia (Box 4.1).

In some contrast to schizophrenia, social withdrawal predominates in autism (Leong and Schilbach 2019). Also, clearly delineated delusions or hallucinations are uncommon in autism (Chandrasekhar et al. 2020). Moreover, there is substantial overlap and comorbidity between autism and other psychiatric conditions beyond schizophrenia (Jokiranta-Olkoniemi et al. 2019; Stralin et al. 2019).

Presently, there is mixed information as to whether—and how often—autism and schizophrenia co-occur, given symptom overlap, particularly in very young children (Chandrasekhar et al. 2020). De Giorgi and colleagues (2019) conducted a systematic review of the prevalence of schizophrenia (they used the term 'non-affective psychosis') in autism. In broadening the criteria to include autism spectrum disorder (ASD), they identified 39 articles describing the overlap between the two conditions. On a more refined evaluation of 14 of these articles that encompassed some 1,700 patients, they arrived at a weighted average prevalence rate of psychosis among autistic individuals of 9.5%. This is clearly above the rate of schizophrenia in the general population, yet it is not so high as other conditions (e.g. depression, OCD) associated with schizophrenia.

Shared neurodevelopmental antecedents between autism and schizophrenia?

Autism is considered a neurodevelopmental disorder (Box 4.2). Heritability studies in autism show a high heritability (Fakhro 2020). More recent molecular genetics studies show an excess of copy number variants (CNVs) in autistic

> **Box 4.2** Brain abnormalities seen in neuroimaging studies of autism
>
> - Enlarged brain, both grey and white matter[*]
> - Selective overenlargement in brain regions[*]
>   - Frontal lobe
>   - Temporal lobe
>   - Occipital lobe
>   - Cerebellum
> - Microstructure dysconnectivity across white matter
> - Demonstrated already in selective brain areas such as corpus callosum
>
> [*]In contrast, these areas are reduced in size in schizophrenia.

individuals (Fakhro 2020; Shaltout et al. 2020). While neither condition has any distinct pattern of CNVs, these micro-deletions and micro-insertions have also been found in schizophrenia. The genetics of autism are complex (Fakhro 2020) and GWAS show aberrant loci and patterns on chromosome 13, 16, 17, 22, and others (Box 4.3). More so than in schizophrenia, these studies have shown associations with genes regulating synaptic proteins and synaptic plasticity. There is also more genetic convergence with schizophrenia. In a recent paper by Gandal and colleagues (2018) there was considerable overlap in the molecular neuropathology between autism and schizophrenia.

Other neurodevelopmental markers are abnormal in both autism and schizophrenia (Kim et al. 2019). Mothers of children with autism have higher rates of obstetric complications, with a trend towards more fetal distress and delivery complications. These features are also found in excess amongst the mothers of individuals with schizophrenia. Improving maternal obstetrical care could reduce autism prevalence (Cheng et al. 2019). Children with autism are more likely than other healthy children to be born in the first 3 months of the year—the so-called

> **Box 4.3** Genetic findings in autism
>
> - Highly heritable (more so than schizophrenia)
> - Excess familial heritability of autism and autistic spectrum disorders
> - Monozygotic twin risk of 80%
> - Dizygotic twin risk of 40%
> - Excess of CNVs
> - Robust and well-replicated association with fragile X syndrome
> - Chromosomes implicated—13, 16, 17, 22
> - Identified selective gene mutations affecting regulation of cell development, synaptic plasticity, tyrosine kinases, cell-adhesion molecules, reelin, and neurexin

season of birth effect. This is also observed in schizophrenia, though at a lower rate of approximately 3.5% of individuals compared with approximately 12% of individuals with autism. Clearly, motor abnormalities are both more prevalent and more pronounced in individuals with autism than they are in people with schizophrenia. The greater prevalence of catatonia in the pre-neuroleptic era, reflecting extreme social withdrawal and marked motor stereotypes, drew attention to the overlap between autism and schizophrenia. Overall, it appears that genetic influences predominate over environmental influences in the pathogenesis of autism (Taylor et al. 2020).

Perhaps the most striking neurobiological finding in autism is that of a larger brain size than normally developing individuals (Girault and Piven 2020). This intriguing finding has been consistently reported in neuroimaging studies in autism. This contrasts with a less pronounced yet quite consistent finding of an approximately 6% reduction in brain size in people with schizophrenia. Additionally, more selective deficits are noted in frontal and temporal lobe regions in schizophrenia, while the occipito-cerebellar region has been consistently implicated in autism. Functional neuroimaging studies show generalized and diffuse hyper-metabolism in autism, with some selective hypo-metabolism in the occipital and cerebellar regions.

Course and treatment divergence between autism and schizophrenia

Both autism and schizophrenia are considered to have some continuum of severity of expression, as manifest in autism spectrum disorder (ASD) and schizophrenia spectrum disorder (SSD) respectively. These do not appear to overlap and/or converge, although both ASD and SSE have high rates of morbid depression. The clinical construct of social anhedonia represents the notable exception where a convergence between autism and schizophrenia is prominent in each condition and may even represent a transdiagnostic state. In the US, the National Institute of Mental Health has developed an Researchers Domain Criteria (RDoC) agenda to try to better understand fundamental constructs that might cut across emotional states and psychiatric conditions (Lindenmayer 2018). Systems for social processes encompass one of the five constructs. Investigating social anhedonia across autism and schizophrenia would be informative.

Treatments for autism and schizophrenia differ greatly. Medications are less often employed in autism and are used for behavioural management and/or depression (Lee et al. 2018). Antidepressants are prescribed more frequently than antipsychotic medications for individuals with autism. Both are associated with a risk of side effects, especially weight gain in young people with autism. Additionally, the multiple comorbidities in autism mean that a wide range of medications are used in such individuals (Lamy and Erickson 2018). Interpersonal and behavioural strategies that are designed to develop and sustain social cues and social awareness and engagement (Lord et al. 2020) are a mainstay of treatment in autism, being much less commonly employed in people with schizophrenia (see Chapter 7).

Conclusions

In conclusion, while early on there was evident sociological uncertainty of the relationship between autism and schizophrenia, it is now more clear that there are many neurobiological similarities between these two conditions. While much research remains to determine the relative contributions of genetic and non-genetic risk factors to each condition, the overall similarities appear at face value to be more expressive of shared neurodevelopmental origins.

REFERENCES

Bhandari R, Paliwal JK, Kuhad A (2020) Neuropsychopathology of autism spectrum disorder: complex interplay of genetic, epigenetic, and environmental factors. Advances in Neurobiology 24: 97–141.

Butlin B, Laws K, Read R, et al. (2019) Concepts of mental disorders in the United Kingdom: similarities and differences between the lay public and psychiatrists. International Journal of Social Psychiatry 65: 507–514.

Chandrasekhar T, Copeland JN, Spanos M, Sikich L (2020) Autism, psychosis, or both? Unraveling complex patient presentations. Child and Adolescent Psychiatric Clinics of North America 29: 1003–1113.

Cheng J, Eskenazi B, Widjaja F, et al. (2019) Improving autism perinatal risk factors: a systematic review. Medical Hypotheses 127: 26–33.

De Giorgi R, De Crescenzo F, D'Alo G, et al. (2019) Prevalence of non-affective psychoses in individuals with autism spectrum disorders: a systematic review. Journal of Clinical Medicine 8: 1304.

Fakhro KA (2020) Genomics of autism. Advances in Neurobiology 24: 83–96.

Gandal MJ, Haney JR, Parikshak NN, Leppa V, et al. (2018) Shared molecular neuropathology across major psychiatric disorders parallels polygenic overlap. Science 359: 693–697.

Girault JB, Piven J (2020) The neurodevelopment of autism from infancy through toddlerhood. Neuroimaging Clinics of North America 30: 97–114.

Jokiranta-Olkoniemi E, Cheslack-Postava K, Joelsson P, et al. (2019) Attention-deficit/hyperactivity disorder and risk for psychiatric and neurodevelopmental disorders in siblings. Psychological Medicine 49: 84–91.

Kim JY, Son, MJ, Son CY, et al. (2019) Environmental risk factors and biomarkers for autism spectrum disorder: an umbrella review of the evidence. Lancet Psychiatry 6: 590–600.

Lamy M, Erickson CA (2018) Pharmacological management of behavioral disturbances in children and adolescents with autism spectrum disorders. Current Problems in Pediatric and Adolescent Health Care 48: 250–264.

Lee ES, Vidal C, Findling FL (2018) A focused review on the treatment of pediatric patients with atypical antipsychotics. Journal of Child and Adolescent Psychopharmacology 28: 582–605.

Leong V, Schilbach L (2019) The promise of two-person neuroscience for developmental psychiatry: using interaction-based sociometrics to identify disorders of social interaction. British Journal of Psychiatry 215: 636–638.

Lindenmayer JP (2018) The NIMH Research Domain Criteria initiative and comorbidity in schizophrenia: research implications. Psychiatric Annals 48: 547–551.

Lord C, Brugha TS, Charman T, et al. (2020) Autism spectrum disorder. Nature Reviews Disease Primers 6: 5.

McCutcheon RA, Marques TR, Howes OD (2020) Schizophrenia—an overview. JAMA Psychiatry 77: 201–210.

Shaltout E, Al-Dewik N, Samara M, et al. (2020) Psychological comorbidities in autism spectrum disorder. Advances in Neurobiology 24: 163–191.

Stralin P, Hetta J (2019) First episode psychosis and comorbid ADHD, autism and intellectual disability. European Psychiatry 55: 18–22.

Taylor MJ, Rosenqvist MA, Larsson H, et al. (2020) Etiology of autism spectrum disorders and autistic traits over time. JAMA Psychiatry e200680, doi: 10.1001/jamapsychiatry.2020.0680.

Zheng A, Zheng P, Zou X (2018) Association between schizophrenia and autism spectrum disorder: a systematic review and meta-analysis. Autism Research 11: 1110–1119.

CHAPTER 4

Personality disorders and schizophrenia

KEY POINTS

- Schizophrenia often manifests early in a person's developmental trajectory and can impact personality development.
- There are neurobiological factors that link schizotypal personality disorder (SPD) and schizophrenia might be considered a 'forme fruste' of schizophrenia.
- People with borderline personality disorder can manifest positive psychotic phenomena that cross-sectionally mimic those of schizophrenia.
- Paranoid personality disorder and psychopathic personality disorder can overlap with schizophrenia, but most people with schizophrenia are not psychopathic.

In Chapter 3, we described the underpinnings of the proposed hierarchical model of mental illness and the emergence of transdiagnostic psychiatry. These constructs are particularly relevant to the consideration of personality disorders as a comorbidity. On one level, the co-existence of personality disorders is antithetical to this hierarchical model, since under this model schizophrenia is considered to be 'at the top of the food chain' and subsumes all other possible diagnoses below (Castle and Buckley 2015; Fusar-Poli 2019). That said, schizophrenia is a condition of pervasive impairments, including that of personality development. This is, of course, particularly so when the onset of psychosis is in youth—early adolescence—which occurs in approximately 25% of individuals (McCutcheon et al. 2020). Moreover, negative symptoms such as avolition, amotivation, anhedonia, and asociality are themselves barriers to the development of the interpersonal relationships that shape personality development (Simonsen and Newton-Howes 2018). Accordingly, consideration of the relationship of personality disorders to the comorbidities of schizophrenia is more selective and circumscribed, as detailed in Boxes 5.1 and 5.2.

Borderline personality disorder and schizophrenia

Borderline personality disorder (BPD) is a pervasive pattern of chaotic interpersonal relationships, anger and agitation, intense feelings of emptiness, instability of mood, and often agitated and self-destructive behaviours. It is important to appreciate that in earlier conceptualizations of mental disorders, BPD was clustered with schizotypal personality disorder (SPD). It had antecedents with earlier

Box 5.1 Personality disorders more associated with schizophrenia

- Borderline
- Paranoid
- Psychopathic
- Schizotypal
- Schizoid

Box 5.2 Personality disorders not usually associated with schizophrenia

- Histrionic
- Narcissistic
- Obsessive compulsive
- Avoidant
- Dependent

constructs characterized by a lack of positive symptoms: 'latent schizophrenia' or 'borderline schizophrenia' or 'pseudo-neurotic schizophrenia'. Josef Parnas, a Danish psychiatrist, is a proponent of this historical antecedent and he has articulated a fundamental relationship between BPD and schizophrenia—one that is encompassed in the model of schizophrenia spectrum disorder (Parnas 2015).

For most patients with BPD, mood disorders, depression, anxiety disorders and substance abuse are the most common and the major comorbidities, and schizophrenia, an especially chronic relapsing illness, is relatively rarely associated with BPD. Having said this, people with BPD are vulnerable to psychotic phenomena that cross-sectionally are similar to the positive symptoms of schizophrenia. For example, studies of auditory hallucinations in individuals with BPD suggest a similar pattern to auditory hallucinations in schizophrenia. Detection of hallucinations is often complicated by reluctance by the patient to describe such 'ego-dystonic' experiences. All that said, individuals with BPD are prone to brief psychotic episodes (Simonsen and Newton-Howes 2018). These are characterized by short-lived hallucinations, paranoid thinking (even to the point of paranoid delusions), and marked anxiety-agitation. These 'micro-psychoses' can occur in individuals with BPD at times of heightened emotional instability (where, under stress, the person in layman's terms 'loses it'). However, brief psychotic episodes that occur in PBD are further complicated as they can occur in the context of use of licit or illicit drugs. In either instance, symptoms subside as the individual becomes less anxious and as the mental state 'reconstitutes'. Antipsychotic medications are usually not indicated in such instances: benzodiazepines are often the more effective option. However, antipsychotics have been studied in BPD to manage chronic instability of mood and anxiety-agitation. There has been some research of a low dose of olanzapine that may demonstrate some small benefit in BPD patients (Camchong et al. 2018). Adverse effects of second-generation antipsychotics, especially weight gain, undermine medication compliance and efficiency particularly in patients with BPD (Koch et al. 2016).

There is no evidence of a 'kindling effect' or successive 'micro-psychoses' that might ultimately devolve to a chronic schizophrenic condition. Similarly, the combination of BPD and cannabis use is no more likely to result in psychosis than is cannabis use alone, though of course there is a heightened rate of cannabis use disorder among BPD patients (Gillespie et al. 2018). A recent study demonstrates similar stress intolerance between people with schizophrenia and people with BPD (Bonfils et al. 2020).

Paranoid personality disorder and schizophrenia

As the name implies, paranoid personality disorder (PPD) is a condition associated with intense and selective mistrust of others and/or situations, paranoid thinking and misinterpretation of events, and associated social isolation (Lee 2017). There can be social and/or occupational impairments, although these are less pronounced than in schizophrenia or other major psychiatric conditions. People with PPD can often be litigious and they can pursue 'redress' for perceived or objectively slight grievances they hold with unshakable conviction. Compared to other psychotic and/or mood disorders, or even compared to other personality disorders, PPD is quite rare. It has high comorbidity with mood disorders, specifically depression, and with anxiety disorders. There is not any notable comorbidity of PPD with schizophrenia and it has not been a feature in recent large epidemiological, descriptive, or genetic studies in schizophrenia. That said, in the 1960s, Sir Martin Roth proposed a 'paranoid spectrum', linking paranoia, PPD and paranoid schizophrenia—especially a late-onset form of paranoid schizophrenia that he termed 'paraphrenia'. Current conceptualizations in geriatric psychiatry recognize the distinction of late-onset schizophrenia, though no link is drawn anymore to PPD and in general this relationship of PPD to schizophrenia is more tenuous than heretofore considered (Lee 2018).

Medication treatment for PPD is limited and adherence to medications is distinctly low due to lack of insight into this condition (Koch et al. 2016).

Psychopathic personality disorder and schizophrenia

Psychopathy, or psychopathic personality disorder, is a relatively common, disabling, and largely intractable personality disorder (Box 5.3).

By definition, psychopathy is preceded by childhood conduct disorder. Although conduct disorder and schizophrenia are different in manifestation, they do share some overlap in risk factors (Abushua'leh and Abu-Akel 2006; Arseneult et al. 2000; Breenan et al. 2000). Social adversity, childhood trauma and childhood sexual abuse are risk factors for both conduct disorder and schizophrenia, though

---

Box 5.3 Diagnostic features of psychopathic personality disorder

* History of conduct disorder
* Disregard for others
* Disregard for legal and social conformations/regulations
* Lack of remorse
* Impulsivity

---

the strength of the associations is far more substantial for conduct disorder (Swanson et al. 2008). Engelstad and colleagues compared childhood trauma and psychopathy in individuals with schizophrenia who had, or had not, committed murder. While psychopathy and childhood trauma were more common among schizophrenia patients who had committed homicide, only psychopathy was a robust predictor of homicidal group status.

Psychopathy is actually not common in individuals with schizophrenia (Castle and Buckley 2015; Fazel et al. 2010). However, to the contrary, there is a broad misperception that it is common, since people with schizophrenia commit more violent actions than the general population (Box 5.4). This association is enshrined in the 'Jekyll and Hyde' misconceptions about schizophrenia, mental illness, and violence. Moreover, and intuitively, psychopathy is overrepresented among patients with schizophrenia who are incarcerated in forensic mental health facilities. Determining intent, disentangling the provocations from psychotic experiences, and discerning the patient's true state of mind at the time of offence are all challenging (O'Reilly et al. 2019; Swanson 2008). This is particularly so because the comorbidity of psychopathy and schizophrenia is inevitability often complicated by comorbid substance abuse and, concomitantly, by non-adherence to anti-psychotic medications (Fazel et al. 2010; Putkonen et al. 2004). This is a large area of forensic psychiatry and the reader is referred to additional information sources regarding this vexing forensic conundrum.

Box 5.4 Violence and schizophrenia: myths that are debunked by 'facts'

* People with schizophrenia are more likely to be victims of violence than perpetrators
* There is a higher rate of violence among people with schizophrenia, compared to the general public
* Violence is more often than not related to untreated, active psychosis
* Violence is often also in the context of active substance abuse
* Violence is more often indiscriminate and directed at relatives or caregivers (close by) rather than at the general public and/or more targeted as in other forms of criminality

---

The comorbidity of psychopathy and schizophrenia raises more fundamental human and societal ethical considerations (Butlin et al. 2019; Cadge et al. 2019). Psychopathy equates in societal terms to 'badness' and schizophrenia equates to 'madness' and there are many divergent viewpoints on these constructs. While cultures and opinions thereupon vary worldwide, in general most societies are ambivalent about how they view mentally ill offenders as either 'bad' or 'mad', or both.

Schizotypal personality disorder, schizoid personality disorder, and schizophrenia

Schizotypal personality disorder (SPD) is slightly more common than schizophrenia (approximately 4% prevalence in the general population) and is in many ways considered a 'form fruste' of schizophrenia. The lay public might refer to this condition as a person having 'a touch of schizophrenia' (Lenzenweger 2018; Parnas 2015). In broad terms, individuals with SPD exhibit social isolation and 'woolly' or hard-to-follow thinking patterns, and they harbour unusual and idiosyncratic ideas. They also exhibit 'negative symptoms' (asociality, anhedonia, amotivation), though these are not as pronounced as in schizophrenia (Kirchner et al. 2018). They are prone to psychotic experiences, both delusions and hallucinations (Box 5.5), but, unlike in BPD, these psychotic experiences are usually not associated with substance misuse, since substance abuse comorbidity is decidedly uncommon in people with SPD. Similarly, and unlike BPD, psychotic experiences in people with SPD may become more frequent and protracted with successive episodes of psychosis. Antipsychotics may help alleviate positive psychotic features and perhaps have some—usually very limited—effect on core negative symptoms, though the evidence for this is sparse (Kirchner et al. 2018; Koch et al. 2016). Schizoid personality disorder also shares some features with SPD, though the overlap with schizophrenia is more with SPD than schizoid personality disorder (Lenzenweger 2018).

In neurobiological terms, SPD is often considered an 'endophenotype' of schizophrenia (Kirchner et al. 2018). Relatives of people with schizophrenia have a higher prevalence of SPD, suggestive of a shared genetic vulnerability. Other

---

Box 5.5 Features of SPD

- Odd, idiosyncratic beliefs
- Referential (but not strictly delusional) thinking
- Odd, idiosyncratic perceptual experiences (but not strictly hallucinations)
- Vague 'woolly thinking' and vague circumstantial speech
- Unusual affect—inappropriate and/or constricted
- Scant social network

Box 5.6 Neurobiological findings in SPD

- Genetic associations (e.g. polymorphisms) and heritability
- Trauma and psychosocial stressors
- Cognitive deficits (similar to schizophrenia though less pronounced)
- Hypo-dopaminergic state—including hypo-frontality on functional neuroimaging
- EEG dyssynchronization
- Subtle eye movement dysfunction and oscillatory imbalance
- Perceptual disturbances including social cognition
- Temporal lobe volume reductions
- Inconsistent findings of frontal lobe grey matter volume reductions
- Structural abnormalities of the temporal lobe as well as more widespread cortical structural dysconnectivity

neurological investigations show similar patterns of disturbances to those seen in people with schizophrenia, albeit in considerably attenuated form (Box 5.6). Aside from SPD, there has been a conspicuous lack of biological research at the interface of personality disorders and schizophrenia.

Other personality disorders and schizophrenia

The associations between schizophrenia reside mostly in 'cluster A' (border-line, schizotypal, paranoid) personality types (as above) and the remaining personality disorders have negligible and/or non-existent associations to schizophrenia (Kirchner et al. 2018). There is no heightened rate of either narcissistic personality disorder or histrionic personality disorder in schizophrenia.

Conclusions

Schizophrenia often manifests early in a person's developmental trajectory and can impact personality development. There are neurobiological factors that link SPD and schizophrenia and SPD might be considered a 'forme fruste' of schizophrenia. People with BPD can manifest positive psychotic phenomena that cross-sectionally mimic those of schizophrenia, but these psychotic experiences tend to be intermittent and stress- or substance-use related, and other features of schizophrenia such as affective restriction are not features of BPD. Paranoid personality disorder and psychopathic personality disorder can overlap with schizophrenia, but most people with schizophrenia are not psychopathic and this is important to consider if we are to reduce the stigma associated with mental illness in general.

REFERENCES

Abushua'leh K, Abu-Akel A (2006) Association of psychopathic traits and symptomatology with violence in patients with schizophrenia. Psychiatry Research 143: 205–211.

Arseneult L, Moffit TE, Caspi A, Taylor PJ, Silva PA (2000) Mental disorders and violence in a total birth cohort: results from the Dunedin Study. Archives of General Psychiatry 57: 979–986.

Bonfils KA, Lysaker PH (2020) Levels of distress tolerance in schizophrenia appear equivalent to those found in borderline personality disorder. Journal of Clinical Psychology doi: 10.1002/jclp.22944.

Breenan PA, Mednick SA, Hodgins S (2000) Major mental disorders and criminal violence in a Danish birth cohort. Archives of General Psychiatry 57: 494–500.

Butlin B, Laws K, Read R, Broome MD, Sharma S (2019) Concepts of mental disorders in the United Kingdom: similarities and differences between the lay public and psychiatrists. International Journal of Social Psychiatry 65: 507–514.

Cadge C, Connor C, Greenfield S (2019) University students' understanding and perceptions of schizophrenia in the UK: a qualitative study. BMJ Open 9: e025813.

Camchong J, Cullen KR, Lim KO, Schulz, SC (2018) Brain metabolism changes in women with BPD undergoing olanzapine treatment. Psychiatry Research Neuroimaging 279: 19–21.

Castle D, Buckley P (2015) Schizophrenia, 2nd edition. Oxford: Oxford University Press.

Fazel S, Buxrud P, Ruchkin V, Grann M (2010) Homicide in discharged patients with schizophrenia and other psychoses: a national case-control study. Schizophrenia Research 123: 263–269.

Fusar-Poli P, Solmi M, Brondino N, et al. (2019) Transdiagnostic psychiatry: a systematic review. World Psychiatry 18: 192–207.

Gillespie NA, Aggen SH, Neale MD, et al. (2018) Associations between personality disorders and cannabis use and cannabis use disorder: a population-based twin study. Addiction 113: 1488–1498.

Kirchner SK, Roeh A, Nolden J, Hasan A (2018) Diagnosis and treatment of schizotypal personality disorder: evidence from a systematic review. NPJ Schizophrenia 4: 20.

Koch J, Modesitt T, Palmer M, et al. (2016) Review of pharmacologic treatment in cluster A personality disorders. Mental Health Clinician 6: 75–81.

Lee R (2017) Mistrustful and misunderstood: a review of paranoid personality disorder. Current Behavioural Neuroscience Reports 4: 151–165.

Lenzenweger MF (2018) Schizotypy, schizotypic psychopathology and schizophrenia. World Psychiatry 17: 25–26.

McCutcheon RA, Marques TR, Howes OD (2020) Schizophrenia—an overview. JAMA Psychiatry 77: 201–210.

O'Reilly K, O'Connell P, O'Sullivan D, et al. (2019) Moral cognition, the missing link between psychotic symptoms and acts of violence: a cross-sectional national forensic cohort study. BMC Psychiatry 9: 408.

Parnas J (2015) Differential diagnosis and current polythetic classification. World Psychiatry 14: 284–287.

Putkonen A, Kotilainen I, Joyal CC, Tiihonen J (2004) Comorbid personality disorders and substance use disorders of mentally ill homicide offenders: a structured clinical study on dual and triple diagnosis. Schizophrenia Bulletin 30: 59–72.

Simonsen E, Newton-Howes G (2018) Personality pathology and schizophrenia. Schizophrenia Bulletin 44: 1180–1184.

Swanson JW, Van Dorn RA, Swartz MS, et al. (2008) Alternative pathways to violence in persons with schizophrenia: the role of childhood antisocial behavior problems. Law and Human Behaviour 32: 228–240.

CHAPTER 5

Generalized anxiety and panic disorder in schizophrenia

KEY POINTS

- Schizophrenia and anxiety disorders occur together much more commonly than would be expected by chance.
- There is evidence that generalized anxiety disorder (GAD) and panic disorder (PD) are particularly prevalent in the prodrome to first episode psychosis.
- Anxiety is also a common early warning sign of psychotic relapse.
- Cognitive models of delusional beliefs feature anxiety.
- Biological explanations for the higher than expected comorbidity include genetic predisposition and the impact of shared environmental factors.
- Treatment of GAD and PD in people with schizophrenia has very little specific direct evidence.
- Cognitive behavioural therapy for psychosis (CBTp) is often focused on reducing delusional distress and anxiety.
- Antidepressant medication is safe to use as adjunct with antipsychotic medication and may be worth an individual patient trial.

There is strong evidence of the common occurrence of panic and generalized anxiety symptoms in schizophrenia, at both the symptom and disorder level. Anxiety symptoms are also prominent in the prodrome of first episode psychosis (FEP) and feature heavily as early warning signs of psychotic relapse. Psychological models of the development of positive symptoms such as persecutory delusions are based on information processing or prediction errors which are related to enhanced 'threat to self' appraisals. Genetic overlaps between risk for schizophrenia and a range of affective and anxiety disorders are becoming clearer with genome-wise association studies, and there is some tantalizing evidence that targeting anxiety may reduce the incidence of psychosis onset or relapse. This all points to anxiety symptoms being an underrecognized area of potentially significant treatment, which may also have wider secondary outcomes. This chapter outlines biological and psychological explanations for the increased incidence of panic and generalized anxiety and provides guidance on its recognition and potential management.

Prevalence of generalized anxiety and panic disorder in schizophrenia

Achim et al. (2009) conducted a systematic review and meta-analysis of all anxiety disorders in schizophrenia, and reported lifetime prevalence rates of up to 24% for generalized anxiety disorder (GAD) and 12% for panic disorder (PD)—considerably higher than the general population (Achim et al. 2009). Rates varied widely, with the level of disorder generally derived from cross-sectional studies that assess symptoms reaching a level of significance for a disorder to be diagnosed. The *lifetime* prevalence of symptoms of anxiety and panic are likely to be much higher still; in one report up to 65% of patients with schizophrenia experienced panic attacks at some point in their illness (Goodwin et al. 2002).

Symptoms of anxiety have been described in patients with schizophrenia for many decades, including in Bleuler's first descriptions of evolving schizophrenia (Buckley et al. 2009). With increasing recognition of a staged model of psychosis and developing mental health disorders in young people (McGorry et al. 2006), psychopathological variability in early phase disorders has also become clear. The ultra-high risk (UHR) phase of psychosis is often accompanied by generalized anxiety and panic: in a recent systematic review, Wilson and colleagues suggest that the prevalence of anxiety in UHR and FEP stages is considerably underestimated (Wilson et al. 2020). Categorical anxiety disorders are likely to represent just one component of a broader continuum of anxiety symptoms that are particularly prevalent in the early stages, when diagnostic fluidity is more apparent; when psychosis is developing in relapse; and when symptoms fluctuate across the course of the disorder.

In terms of PD specifically, Hofmann and colleagues (2000) put forward a number of hypotheses to explain the co-occurrence with schizophrenia, including that autonomic hyperactivity associated with panic may serve as a stressor to induce or exacerbate psychotic symptoms, again reinforcing the idea that anxiety symptoms may be most relevant in the development and maintenance of psychopathology (Hofmann et al. 2000).

In psychotic relapse, the identification of early warning signs has become established practice, with their successful identification linked with the ability of individuals and their clinical teams to alter treatment plans, reduce environmental pressures, or alter pharmacological regimes prior to the full manifestation of psychotic relapse (Birchwood et al. 2000). Early warning signs are now recognized to include both psychosis precursors such as thought disorganization, low-level paranoid ideation and social withdrawal, and 'neurosis' factors, such as anxiety and depression (Bustillo et al. 1995). Norman and Malla (1995) highlighted the importance of such non-psychotic symptoms, suggesting that they may be useful to identify psychotic relapse and also they are related to early and subtle signs of psychosis (Norman and Malla 1995).

What are the causes of an increased occurrence of anxiety in schizophrenia?

If anxiety symptoms are present in UHR phases, and prior to psychotic relapse, there follows a likelihood that they may be a precursor to schizophrenia. Anxiety symptoms are prominent in cognitive models of positive symptoms of psychosis. Population-based studies such as the Avon Longitudinal Study of Parents and Children (ALSPAC) indicate that young people with high levels of anxiety are more likely to experience psychotic symptoms, with symptoms representing a manifestation of a unitary, latent continuum of common mental disorder, with psychotic experiences conveying information about the more severe end (Stochl et al. 2015). This conclusion is in keeping with the hierarchical model outlined in Chapter 3, whereby in the presence a more severe illness, symptoms common in other 'less severe' syndromes such as GAD are to be expected (Foulds and Bedford 1975). As PD is also common in the UHR phase (Rapp et al. 2012; Tien and Eaton 1992), people with panic symptoms are unsurprisingly more likely to seek help early than those without panic disorder (Goodwin et al. 2002).

The ALSPAC cohort also demonstrated that a high polygenic risk score for schizophrenia is expressed in the increased likelihood of broadly occurring anxiety symptoms as well as positive symptoms of psychosis (Jones et al. 2016). Similarly, the Edinburgh High Risk Study of schizophrenia showed that anxiety and mood symptoms preceded the onset of psychotic symptoms in those who went on to develop a psychotic disorder (Owens et al. 2005). Understanding causal mechanisms and developing targeted interventions would be needed to elucidate whether the common symptoms of anxiety are simply harbingers of more severe psychopathology or are indeed causally related to schizophrenia. Longitudinal studies demonstrating the temporal relationship between GAD and PD and risk for schizophrenia give important information. However, psychosis itself is a stressful life event for many people, and GAD and PD are equally likely to be precipitated by this experience; therefore models should take into account the anxiety-provoking consequences of psychosis, as well as how these experiences may precipitate psychotic relapse.

Cognitive models of generalized anxiety and psychosis

A number of psychosis risk factors—including minority status, childhood trauma, and migration—increase the risk of anxiety disorders. These non-specific factors of poor mental health may also be precursors to substance misuse, depression, and other mental health outcomes. However, heightened anxiety can bias both perception and cognition and may contribute to the development of positive psychotic symptoms and their perceived distress and need for care.

Freeman and Garety have developed robust models of persecutory delusions based on the premise that worry and the process of anxiety are essential for the development and maintenance of delusional distress (Freeman and Garety 2003;

Garety and Freeman 1999). General anxiety, worry, and meta-cognitive processes were found to be related to the development of delusional thinking. The content of persecutory delusions is conceptualized as threat beliefs, and then maintained by confirmatory 'evidence', with heightened threat to self-appraisals not allowing disconfirmatory evidence to enter the equation. However, in contrast to individuals with GAD and no psychosis, psychotic individuals are more likely to look out for threat (Freeman et al. 2002), whilst worry in people with persecutory delusions is associated with more perseverative thinking, catastrophizing, and intolerance of uncertainty (Startup et al. 2007). These models form the basis of cognitive behavioural therapy for psychosis (CBTp). Although not without controversy (Jauhar et al. 2019), evidence suggests CBTp can be effective in terms of reducing delusional distress and improving acute symptoms for transitory periods (Lewis et al. 2002), and although studies that make no attempt to mask group allocation are likely to inflate effect sizes, positive results appear to be seen to some extent also for secondary outcomes, including anxiety (Wykes et al. 2008).

In terms of auditory hallucinations, distress and anxiety are strongly linked with the experience of anomalous perceptions and the need for care. Clinical voice hearers are more likely to report negative beliefs, worry, and lack of control than non-clinical voice hearers and it may be the distress itself leads to help-seeking (Hill and Linden 2013). Woods et al. (2015) reported that around a third of voice hearers have anxiety as a core part of the experience (Woods et al. 2015). A systematic review also highlighted the high frequency of insecure or anxious attachment in people who manifest psychotic symptoms: insecurely attached individuals were more likely to develop maladaptive coping strategies for processing social information, mentalization, and developing social relationships (Korver-Nieberg et al. 2014). Social isolation may be a pathway to anxiety-driven psychotic phenomenology in vulnerable individuals.

Biological models

As detailed in Chapter 1, schizophrenia is a highly heritable condition, with genomic factors explaining around 65–80% of the variance in risk (Purcell et al. 2009; Sullivan et al. 2012). However, this risk is shared amongst many common risk alleles, each of small effect; combined together these risk alleles at an individual level can be used to generate a polygenic risk score (PRS). Schizophrenia PRSs correlate with schizophrenia status, but also with other disorders including bipolar disorder and depression (Richards et al. 2019). Regarding anxiety disorders, Jones et al. (2016), using the ALSPAC cohort, demonstrated that PRS was associated with anxiety and negative symptoms in adolescents (Jones et al. 2016); and other researchers using the same cohort showed that the PRS for schizophrenia conferred risk specifically for GAD and PD, and this extended into adulthood as well as adolescence (Richards et al. 2019). This has been replicated in a separate cohort, from New Zealand, with odds ratios (ORs) for PRS for schizophrenia and GAD being 1.5 and for PD 1.3. These findings suggest the co-occurrence of schizophrenia and GAD/PD is driven at least in part by common biological antecedents.

Increased release of presynaptic dopamine remains the prevailing model of positive symptoms of schizophrenia (Howes and Kapur 2009), compatible with the efficacy of antipsychotic medications that act as dopamine antagonists. However, it should be noted that antipsychotic medications when first produced were labelled as 'major tranquillizers' and the vast majority of first and second generation antipsychotics have sedative effects secondary to histaminergic function. Thus anxiety, in the broadest sense, may well be treated serendipitously when positive symptoms are targeted. Whilst dopamine may be a final common pathway for positive symptoms, other non-dopaminergic pathways are active and may well be relevant when considering comorbidities, including glutaminergic and immune mechanisms (see Chapter 3). Thus, understanding and recognizing GAD and PD comorbidity is important not only for treating an underrecognized comorbidity, but also for driving the development of novel treatments.

Recognition of GAD and PD in schizophrenia

Recognition of GAD and PD in people with schizophrenia requires careful consideration and elucidation of positive, negative, and general symptoms (Box 6.1). Anxiety can present as secondary to explicit threat from perceived persecutors as part of fully formed delusions or be present in the prodrome. It can also manifest as part the phenomenology associated with the development of primary delusions, manifesting as uncomfortable feelings or delusional mood. Negative symptoms such as amotivation and avoidance may be secondary to avoidance of anxiety-provoking situations. GAD and PD may be a reactive manifestation to external circumstances or as a discrete comorbid condition. In all scenarios, they

---

Box 6.1 Features of schizophrenia comorbid with GAD and PD

- GAD and PD can occur secondary to positive symptoms, as a manifestation of the threat from persecutors or coercive treatment
- GAD and PD can be prodromal symptoms in first episode and psychotic relapse
- GAD and PD may be directly related to delusional distress and malevolent or threatening auditory hallucinations
- Schizophrenia patients with comorbid GAD and PD may have greater insight
- GAD and PD comorbidity can have significant detrimental effect on prognosis, functional recovery, and quality of life
- PD may be more common in those with paranoid schizophrenia rather than other subtypes

can have profound negative effects on prognosis, functional recovery, and quality of life (Buckley et al. 2009).

Some evidence suggests that patients with prominent paranoid symptoms are more likely to experience GAD and PD (Savitz et al. 2011). This is in keeping with the cognitive models discussed above. Schizophrenia patients with GAD and PD comorbidity may also have generally higher levels of cognitive functioning, including verbal reasoning (Rapp et al. 2012), and have increased levels of insight compared to patients with schizophrenia without this comorbidity (Buckley et al. 2008). However, patients with comorbid GAD and PD also are more likely to have other comorbidities, such as depression and substance misuse (Goodwin et al. 2003).

Management of GAD and PD in schizophrenia

Management of GAD and PD in schizophrenia needs to take into account the likely underlying cause, i.e. whether anxiety is related to undertreated positive symptoms or is identified as an early warning sign of psychotic relapse. Careful review of symptoms and their development and weight in the overall presentation is required. Management thereafter can be grouped into psychological interventions and pharmacological, taken largely wholesale from effective treatment strategies for anxiety disorders outside of schizophrenia comorbidity. We are aware of very few specific clinical intervention trials for GAD and PD comorbid with schizophrenia.

As outlined above, cognitive models of the development and maintenance of delusional beliefs focus heavily on the presence of, and relationship to, delusional distress. Thus, some evidence can be extrapolated from CBTp to inform interventions addressing comorbid anxiety symptoms. CBTp aims to reduce catastrophic appraisals and related distress and includes the adoption of coping strategies that will reduce anxiety associated with positive symptoms. Strategies include behavioural rehearsal and the reversal of avoidance (or safety behaviours) as common approaches (Wykes et al. 2007). CBTp trials have mostly targeted positive symptoms and/or transition to psychosis as primary outcomes, albeit some also report secondary effects on affective symptoms. Most larger higher-quality trials find effects for CBTp on positive symptoms and/or relapse prevention in the small effect size range (Jauhar et al. 2014). Some evidence suggests CBTp has an effect on anxiety symptoms, although evidence for this exists primarily from trials on social anxiety (Kingsep et al. 2003). Hofmann et al. reported a case series of CBT for panic disorder modified for schizophrenia, building on evidence that CBT is most effective for PD even when compared to pharmacological treatment, and has smaller drop-out rates (Hofmann et al. 2000).

In terms of pharmacological management, choice of antipsychotic medication and adjunctive medication should be considered. There is some evidence that anxiety symptoms are more prevalent in patients who are coprescribed multiple psychotropic medication (Howells et al. 2017) and mixed evidence that antipsychotic medication may increase or decrease anxiety (Buckley et al. 2009). Exacerbation of extrapyramidal side effects and new presentation of akathisia, with subjective distress and restlessness, needs careful assessment. First generation antipsychotic medication (e.g. haloperidol) may be associated with an increase in anxiety, whereas there is evidence that some second generation antipsychotics with more sedative properties may be useful as anxiolytics; this is usually off label and without direct trial evidence. The strongest evidence for antipsychotic effectiveness in GAD without schizophrenia comorbidity is for the use of quetiapine in treatment of acute anxiety (Baldwin et al. 2011, 2014).

Antidepressant medications, particularly selective serotonin reuptake inhibitors (SSRIs), are the first line pharmacological indication for the treatment of GAD and PD without schizophrenia comorbidity; however, there have been no direct trials of antidepressant medication for the treatment indication. In a systematic review of the treatment of anxiety disorders in schizophrenia, the majority of studies were in OCD (see Chapter 8), with PD literature primarily consisting of case reports (Braga et al. 2013).

SSRIs and other antidepressant medication may be safely co-prescribed in adjunct to antipsychotic medication, with appropriate monitoring for the increased potential side effects, including prolongation of QTc interval. In a large population-based sample, Tiihonen and colleagues reported that adjunctive prescribing of antidepressants with antipsychotic medication was associated with a reduced all-cause mortality and with no increase in cardiovascular events (Tiihonen et al. 2012). Helfer reported that adding an antidepressant to an antipsychotic regimen did not increase rates of relapse in psychosis and did not increase the rate of drop-out (Helfer et al. 2016). Having said this, specific side effects and interaction effects need to be borne in mind when co-prescribing: the reader is referred to Chapter 10 for further details. Box 6.2 provides an overview of treatment approaches to GAD and PD in people with schizophrenia.

Box 6.2 Treatment of schizophrenia comorbid with GAD and PD

- Give careful consideration to the possibility that symptoms of GAD and PD may be early warning signs of psychotic relapse
- CBT may be best focused on delusional distress, panic, and anxiety rather than positive symptoms, but evidence is lacking
- Measures to increase insight need to be used with awareness that this may also increase anxiety (and depression: see Chapter 10)
- Consider choice of antipsychotic medication; assess carefully for akathisia
- Antidepressant medication (SSRIs) can be considered in individual patient trials and should be stopped if there is no added benefit
- Benzodiazepines should generally be avoided in all but very short-term use (days to weeks)

Conclusions

GAD and PD are significant yet underrecognized comorbidities that affect high numbers of patients with schizophrenia. For some they may have a causal role in the development and maintenance of positive symptoms of psychosis, and/or herald psychotic relapse. Recognition of GAD and PD in schizophrenia takes skill, careful consideration, and a good therapeutic relationship to elucidate complex psychopathology. More treatment and prevention trials are needed to understand better the potential benefits that increased focus on this area of unmet need may bring.

REFERENCES

Achim AM, Maziade M, Raymond É, et al. (2009) How prevalent are anxiety disorders in schizophrenia? A meta-analysis and critical review on a significant association. Schizophrenia Bulletin 37: 811–821.

Baldwin DS, Waldman S, Allgulander C (2011) Evidence-based pharmacological treatment of generalized anxiety disorder. International Journal of Neuropsychopharmacology 14: 697–710.

Baldwin DS, Anderson IM, Nutt DJ, et al. (2014) Evidence-based pharmacological treatment of anxiety disorders, post-traumatic stress disorder and obsessive-compulsive disorder: a revision of the 2005 guidelines from the British Association for Psychopharmacology. Journal of Psychopharmacology 28: 403–439.

Birchwood M, Spencer E, McGovern D (2000) Schizophrenia: early warning signs. Advances in Psychiatric Treatment 6: 93–101.

Braga RJ, Reynolds GP, Siris SG (2013) Anxiety comorbidity in schizophrenia. Psychiatry Research 210: 1–7.

Buckley PF, Miller BJ, Lehrer DS, Castle DJ (2009) Psychiatric comorbidities and schizophrenia. Schizophrenia Bulletin 35: 383–402.

Bustillo J, Buchanan R, Carpenter WT Jr (1995) Prodromal symptoms vs. early warning signs and clinical action in schizophrenia. Schizophrenia Bulletin 21: 553–559.

Foulds GA, Bedford A (1975) Hierarchy of classes of personal illness. Psychological Medicine 5: 181–192.

Freeman D, Garety PA (2003) Connecting neurosis and psychosis: the direct influence of emotion on delusions and hallucinations. Behaviour Research and Therapy 41: 923–947.

Freeman D, Garety PA, Kuipers E, et al. (2002) A cognitive model of persecutory delusions. British Journal of Clinical Psychology 41: 331–347.

Garety PA, Freeman D (1999) Cognitive approaches to delusions: a critical review of theories and evidence. British Journal of Clinical Psychology 38: 113–154.

Goodwin R, Lyons JS, McMally RJ (2002) Panic attacks in schizophrenia. Schizophrenia Research 58: 213–220.

Goodwin RD, Amador XF, Malaspina D, et al. (2003) Anxiety and substance use comorbidity among inpatients with schizophrenia. Schizophrenia Research 61: 89–95.

Helfer B, Samara MT, Huhn M, et al. (2016) Efficacy and safety of antidepressants added to antipsychotics for schizophrenia: a systematic review and meta-analysis. American Journal of Psychiatry 173: 876–886.

Hill K, Linden DE (2013) Hallucinatory experiences in non-clinical populations. In: Thomas P, Jardri R, Pins D, Cachia A (eds) The Neuroscience of Hallucinations. New York: Springer.

Hofmann SG, Bufka LF, Brady SM, et al. (2000) Cognitive-behavioral treatment of panic in patients with schizophrenia: preliminary findings. Journal of Cognitive Psychotherapy 14: 381.

Howells FM, Kingdon DG, Baldwin DS (2017) Current and potential pharmacological and psychosocial interventions for anxiety symptoms and disorders in patients with schizophrenia: structured review. Human Psychopharmacology: Clinical and Experimental 32: e2628.

Howes OD, Kapur S (2009) The dopamine hypothesis of schizophrenia: version III—the final common pathway. Schizophrenia Bulletin 35: 549–562.

Jauhar S, McKenna P, Radua J, et al. (2014) Cognitive-behavioural therapy for the symptoms of schizophrenia: systematic review and meta-analysis with examination of potential bias. British Journal of Psychiatry 204: 20–29.

Jauhar S, Laws K, McKenna P (2019) CBT for schizophrenia: a critical viewpoint. Psychological Medicine 49: 1233–1236.

Jones HJ, Stergiakouli E, Tansey KE, et al (2016) Phenotypic manifestation of genetic risk for schizophrenia during adolescence in the general population. JAMA Psychiatry 73: 221–228.

Khandaker GM, Zammit S, Burgess S, et al. (2018) Association between a functional interleukin 6 receptor genetic variant and risk of depression and psychosis in a population-based birth cohort. Brain, Behavior and Immunity 69: 264–272.

Kingsep P, Nathan P, Castle D (2003) Cognitive behavioural group treatment for social anxiety in schizophrenia. Schizophrenia Research 63: 121–129.

Korver-Nieberg N, Berry K, Meijer CJ, DeHaan L (2014) Adult attachment and psychotic phenomenology in clinical and non-clinical samples: a systematic review. Psychology and Psychotherapy: Theory, Research and Practice 87: 127–154.

Lewis S, Tarrier N, Haddock G, et al. (2002) Randomised controlled trial of cognitive-behavioural therapy in early schizophrenia: acute-phase outcomes. British Journal of Psychiatry 181: s91–s97.

McGorry PD, Hickie IB, Yung AR, et al. (2006) Clinical staging of psychiatric disorders: a heuristic framework for choosing earlier, safer and more effective interventions. Australian and New Zealand Journal of Psychiatry 40: 616–622.

Norman RM, Malla AK (1995) Prodromal symptoms of relapse in schizophrenia: a review. Schizophrenia Bulletin 21: 527–539.

Owens DC, Miller P, Lawrie SM, Johnstone EC (2005) Pathogenesis of schizophrenia: a psychopathological perspective. British Journal of Psychiatry 186: 386–393.

Purcell SM, Wray NR, Stone JL, et al. (2009) Common polygenic variation contributes to risk of schizophrenia and bipolar disorder. Nature 460: 748–752.

Rapp EK, White-Ajmani ML, Antonius D, et al. (2012) Schizophrenia comorbid with panic disorder: evidence for distinct cognitive profiles. Psychiatry Research 197: 206–211.

Richards A, Horwood J, Boden J, et al. (2019) Associations between schizophrenia genetic risk, anxiety disorders and manic/hypomanic episode in a longitudinal population cohort study. British Journal of Psychiatry 214: 96–102.

Savitz AJ, Kahn TA, McGovern KE, Kahn JP (2011) Carbon dioxide induction of panic anxiety in schizophrenia with auditory hallucinations. Psychiatry Research 189: 38–42.

Startup H, Freeman D, Garety PA (2007) Persecutory delusions and catastrophic worry in psychosis: developing the understanding of delusion distress and persistence. Behaviour Research and Therapy 45: 523–537.

Stochl J, Khandaker G, Lewis G, et al. (2015) Mood, anxiety and psychotic phenomena measure a common psychopathological factor. Psychological Medicine 45: 1483–1493.

Sullivan PF, Daly MJ, O'Donovan M (2012) Genetic architectures of psychiatric disorders: the emerging picture and its implications. Nature Reviews Genetics 13: 537.

Tien AY, Eaton WW (1992) Psychopathologic precursors and sociodemographic risk factors for the schizophrenia syndrome. Archives of General Psychiatry 49: 37–46.

Tiihonen J, Suokas JT, Suvisaari JM, et al. (2012) Polypharmacy with antipsychotics, antidepressants, or benzodiazepines and mortality in schizophrenia. Archives of General Psychiatry 69: 476–483.

Upthegrove R, Manzanares-Teson N, Barnes NM (2014) Cytokine function in medication-naive first episode psychosis: a systematic review and meta-analysis. Schizophrenia Research 155: 101–108.

Wilson RS, Yung AR, Morrison AP (2020) Comorbidity rates of depression and anxiety in first episode psychosis: a systematic review and meta-analysis. Schizophrenia Research 216: 322–329.

Woods A, Jones N, Alderson-Day B, et al. (2015) Experiences of hearing voices: analysis of a novel phenomenological survey. Lancet Psychiatry 2: 323–331.

Wykes T, Steel C, Everitt B, Tarrier N (2007) Cognitive behavior therapy for schizophrenia: effect sizes, clinical models, and methodological rigor. Schizophrenia Bulletin 34: 523–537.

CHAPTER 6

CHAPTER 7

Social anxiety disorder and schizophrenia

> **KEY POINTS**
>
> * Social anxiety disorder affects around 1 in 5 people with schizophrenia.
> * Comorbid social anxiety disorder is associated with numerous adverse consequences for people with schizophrenia, including social isolation, reduced employment rates, and alcohol use.
> * It is important to differentiate social anxiety from negative or positive symptoms of schizophrenia by asking about the cognitions (i.e. fear of negative evaluation by others).
> * Social anxiety in people with schizophrenia can be effectively treated, notably using cognitive behavioural group therapy.

The importance of recognizing social anxiety disorder comorbidity in schizophrenia rests largely in the fact that once recognized, it can be effectively treated and consequently improve the social integration and overall life enjoyment of the individual. A common trap is to assume that social withdrawal in someone with schizophrenia is a consequence of negative symptoms of schizophrenia: that might be the case, but it also might well be that the individual is experiencing anxiety about socializing. The tendency to interpret the behaviours of people as consequent upon their diagnostic label is what Thomas Scheff (1974) called 'labelling theory'. It does people a dis-service and results in specific problems not being adequately addressed (see also Chapter 3). Thus, this chapter explores the rates of social anxiety disorder in people with schizophrenia; provides clinical tips as to how to delineate social anxiety from psychotic symptoms; addresses other important comorbidities; and outlines a treatment approach to managing social anxiety symptoms in people with schizophrenia.

How common is social anxiety disorder in people with schizophrenia?

The prevalence of social anxiety disorder in people with schizophrenia has been the subject of a recent systematic review and meta-analysis (McEnery et al. 2019). The review encompassed 92,522 people from 25 studies conducted across 13 countries. The pooled prevalence rate for social anxiety disorder was 21% (16–26%). Rates were overall higher in outpatient compared to inpatient samples: 25% (19–31%) in the former and 9% (7–12%) in the latter.

In terms of illness phase, a number of studies have specifically assessed rates of social anxiety disorder in first episode psychosis. An early study by Michail and Birchwood (2009) reported a rate of 25% in 80 people with early psychosis; a further 11.6% were reported to have severe social difficulties but did not meet diagnostic criteria (ICD-10) for social anxiety disorder.

Diagnosing social anxiety disorder in people with schizophrenia

Perhaps most important in the evaluation of social anxiety disorder in people with schizophrenia is to ensure the correct clinical questions are asked, and not pre-judging behaviours as 'due to' the schizophrenia itself. As outlined above, negative symptoms in particular can result in social withdrawal; and positive symptoms can cause the individual substantial distress and lead them to avoid social situations in which they feel threatened or at risk in some way. As detailed in Chapter 10, depression is common amongst people with schizophrenia and is also a contributor to social withdrawal.

Thus, the key differentiating questions that need to be asked are those that interrogate the core behaviours and cognitions associated with social anxiety disorder, notably fear of negative evaluation by others and avoidance behaviours. Enquiry should be made about specific cognitions in social situations as well as any autonomic symptoms. It can be useful to ask the individual to think about the last time they were in a social setting and what they felt and thought at the time. Exploring the cognitions can be instructive in differentiating psychotic beliefs (e.g. being persecuted or spied upon, or having referential ideation) from fear of embarrassment in social anxiety disorder. Anticipatory anxiety prior to social engagements is very common in people with social anxiety disorder. Unlike with negative symptoms, the person desires to socialize but feels too anxious; people with predominant negative symptoms simply don't have the wherewithal to socialize and it is not really on their agenda. People with more prominent positive symptoms will often have a more specific delusional set of beliefs that lead them to avoid socializing. Additionally, it is generally the case that social anxiety concerns are seen by the individual as excessive, whereas delusional beliefs are not amenable to question.

A number of different assessment schedules have been used in studies of social anxiety in schizophrenia. There is no absolute 'gold standard' scale in this regard, but the Liebowitz Social Anxiety Scale (LSAS) (Liebowitz 1987) has been widely used and the domains covered seem readily applicable in people with schizophrenia in whom social anxiety disorder is suspected (see Box 7.1).

Box 7.1 Synopsis of domains encompassed by the LSAS

Public performance factor

- Performing or giving a talk to an audience
- Being the centre of attention
- Reporting to a group
- Speaking up at a meeting
- Entering a room where others are seated
- Engaging with small groups
- Attending a party
- Being observed whilst working
- Trying to pick someone up

Social interaction factor

- Making direct eye contact with someone not well known to you
- Talking to people not well known to you
- Calling someone not well known to you
- Meeting strangers
- Expressing disagreement/disapproval to people not well known to you
- Returning items to a shop
- Resisting a salesperson
- Giving a party

Observation factor

- Being scrutinized whilst writing
- Eating in public
- Drinking with others in public
- Urinating in a public facility
- Telephoning in public

Adapted with permission from Liebowitz, M. Social phobia. *Modern Problems of Pharmacopsychiatry*, 22: 141–173. Copyright 1987 by S. Karger AG.

A cut-off score of 29/30 has been applied in schizophrenia samples (Lowengrub et al. 2015).

Pallanti et al. (2006) suggest that a clinician administer the social anxiety rating scale as well as other psychopathology scales as this allows a weighing of psychotic vs. anxiety symptoms and determination of any interactions between these. Having said this, Romm et al. (2011) explored the factor structure of social anxiety disorder based on self-report with the LSAS in 144 people with early psychosis and determined a three-factor structure, viz public performance, social interaction and observation (see Box 7.1). These factors are compatible with findings from people with social anxiety disorder who do not have schizophrenia and suggest utility of the self-report LSAS in this population.

What other comorbidities need to be considered?

Depression commonly accompanies social anxiety in people in the general population and is arguably even more problematic for people with schizophrenia. Part of the explanation is that social anxiety leads to social isolation and thus precludes social integration and connection. This fuels 'self-stigma' and is also an additional barrier to achieving educational or vocational success. This feeds a cycle of isolation, poverty, and lack of meaning that can be so demoralizing for people with schizophrenia (see Chapter 10).

Obesity and concomitant *body image concerns* are unfortunately very common amongst people with schizophrenia. This can be another contributor to social avoidance, with shame about physical appearance feeding social anxiety and the belief that people are judging them negatively. This results in more restricted lifestyles and lack of exercise, which in turn exacerbates physical health problems.

It is very common for people with social anxiety to use *alcohol* as a way of coping with the anxiety that socializing carries with it. Alcohol as a 'social lubricant' is so widely accepted in most societies and alcohol is so readily available that people often do not realise that excessive use carries profound potential negative consequences for both their physical and mental health. For people with schizophrenia there are added burdens related to cost of alcohol as a proportional expense for people who are often on social benefits; interactions with prescribed drugs; physical health consequences including obesity; and mental health implications, notably sleep disturbance and worsening of anxiety symptoms and depressed mood. For a detailed outline of the assessment and management of alcohol and other drug comorbidities in people with schizophrenia the reader is referred to Chapters 11 and 12.

Aside from these factors, a number of studies have reported that people with schizophrenia who have comorbid social anxiety exhibit particularly severe psychotic symptoms, across a number of domains (see Box 7.2). As outlined above, this should not lead to the assumption that the social anxiety symptoms are simply reflective of severe psychosis. Or course, an assessment of the reasons for social avoidance needs to build in an understanding of potential drivers in terms of both positive and negative psychotic symptoms, but the presence of such symptoms should not preclude trying to address the social anxiety directly.

Treating social anxiety disorder in people with schizophrenia

Psychological approaches to treatment

Cognitive behavioural therapy (CBT) has been effectively deployed to target social anxiety symptoms in people with schizophrenia. For example, Kingsep and colleagues (2003) performed a randomized controlled trial of group-based CBT (waitlist control) with 41 people (33 completers) with schizophrenia who also

Box 7.2 Associated features of schizophrenia and social anxiety

- Depression
- Suicidality
- Alcohol and other drug use
- Greater burden of positive psychotic symptoms
- More persecutory beliefs
- Bizarre behaviour
- Social exclusion
- Reduced quality of life
- Unemployment

Source: Data from Pallanti, S., Quercioli, L., Hollander, E. (2004) Social anxiety in outpatients with schizophrenia: a relevant cause of disability. *American Journal of Psychiatry*, 161: 53–58; Lowengrub, K.M., Stryer, R., Birger, M., Iancu, I. (2015) Social anxiety disorder comorbid with schizophrenia: the importance of screening for this underrecognised and undertreated condition. *Israeli Journal of Psychiatry and Related Sciences*, 52: 40–46; McEnery, C., Lim, M.H., Tremain, H., et al. (2019) Prevalence rate of social anxiety disorder in individuals with a psychotic disorder: a systematic review and meta-analysis. *Schizophrenia Research*, 208: 25–33.

met criteria for social anxiety disorder. The content of the 12-session programme is summarized in Box 7.3. The general principles encompassed:

- Psycho-education
- Exposure simulations
- Cognitive restructuring
- Role play
- Inter-session homework.

The intervention group showed highly significant reductions in social interaction anxiety and concomitant improvements in quality and enjoyment of life. Importantly there was no worsening of psychotic symptoms. The main adaptation from such a programme employed for people without schizophrenia lay in the case managers working with the participants between group sessions to model social behaviours and support them in undertaking their exposure homework.

Social skills training

There is a very large literature on social skills training as it pertains to people with schizophrenia (see Box 7.4 for a summary of techniques). The intent here is more focused on teaching people to develop social skills, rather than specific attention to social anxiety symptoms. Having said this, it seems obvious that if people gain confidence and adeptness with social niceties, their interaction with others will be made easier and anxiety should be reduced. Wallace et al. (1980), in a review and

Box 7.3 Synopsis of session-by-session content of CBT program for social anxiety in schizophrenia

- Session 1: Introduction: group context, general psychoeducation, and addressing motivation to change
- Session 2: Introduce concepts of anxiety monitoring and thought monitoring
- Session 3: Use of diaphragmatic breathing; linkage between actions, thoughts, and feelings; and identifying unhelpful thoughts
- Session 4: Challenging unhelpful thoughts
- Session 5: Exposure paradigm and hierarchical approach to facing feared situations
- Session 6: Explain 'covert' relaxation techniques
- Session 7: Role play within the group
- Session 8: Extend and expand role play
- Session 9: Use of 'coping cards'
- Session 10: Discuss relapse prevention strategies
- Session 11: Program review and further role pay
- Session 12: Group review and celebration

Adapted with permission from Kingsep, P., Nathan, P., Castle, D. Cognitive behavioural group treatment for social anxiety in schizophrenia. *Schizophrenia Research*, 63: 121–129. Copyright © 2003 Elsevier Science B.V. All rights reserved.

critique of this area, concluded that social skills training does result in improvements in measures of social anxiety and discomfort, but that these gains do not generalize across other social scenarios or result in improved quality of life. Having said this, some of the topographical strategies and skill-building techniques seem intuitively to have utility in enhancing self-confidence and social adeptness in people with schizophrenia who have social disabilities. Research specifically integrating these parameters into programmes addressing social anxiety in people with schizophrenia is warranted.

Box 7.4 Summary of elements of social skills training

- Shaping
- Positive reinforcement
- Negative reinforcement
- Prompting
- Modelling
- Behaviour rehearsal

Source: Data from Wallace, C.J., Nelson, C.J., Liberman, R.P., et al. (1980) A review and critique of social skills training with schizophrenic patients. *Schizophrenia Bulletin*, 6: 42–63.

Pharmacological approaches to treatment

There is scant research on pharmacological treatments for social anxiety disorder in people with schizophrenia. Indeed, a psychotic illness would be an exclusion criterion for most trials of medications for social anxiety disorder. Hence, we need to draw on the available literature on social anxiety disorder per se to inform pharmacological management of social anxiety in schizophrenia. There is good evidence for a number of selective serotonin reuptake inhibitors (SSRIs) and serotonin noradrenaline reuptake inhibitors (SNRIs), as well as for the reversible inhibitors of monoamine oxidase A (RIMA), moclobemide, for social anxiety disorder (Bandelow et al. 2017). The use of such agents in people taking concomitant antipsychotics needs to consider drug–drug interactions, as well as cumulative side effects and a possibility of worsening of psychotic symptoms with some agents. For a detailed discussion of these factors see Chapter 10.

A relatively novel approach to the treatment of social anxiety disorder is the use of the neuropeptide oxytocin, although results of clinical trials have been rather equivocal (e.g. Guastella et al. 2009). Oxytocin has also been investigated in schizophrenia, to try to promote pro-social behaviours, but not specifically in people with comorbid social anxiety disorder. For example, Halverson et al. (2019) performed a randomized controlled trial of 24 IU of oxytocin intranasally vs. placebo in 68 people with schizophrenia or schizoaffective disorder, targeting empathy and introspective accuracy, as well as self-reported social anxiety (measured with the LSAS). Outcomes at 12 weeks revealed only a very small effect of oxytocin on a measure of perspective-taking and no significant reduction in self-reported social anxiety symptoms. Whether a schizophrenia group selected for comorbid social anxiety disorder would show benefit from oxytocin remains to be tested.

Conclusions

Social anxiety disorder is a common comorbid condition in people with schizophrenia. It is often missed in clinical practice, with clinicians tending to assume that lack of socialization is due to the negative symptoms of schizophrenia or that the individual is responding to positive psychotic symptoms. Specific questioning regarding the core cognitions associated with social anxiety disorder (i.e. fear of negative evaluation by others) is required to delineate the disorder. Treatment with cognitive behavioural techniques (preferably group-based) can be effective in ameliorating the social anxiety symptoms and improving social integration and quality of life. Certain antidepressant drugs can also be effective, but side effects, drug–drug interactions, and potential for worsening of psychotic symptoms need to be weighed before adding them to antipsychotic medication regimes.

REFERENCES

Bandelow B, Michaelis S, Wedekind D (2017) Treatment of anxiety. Dialogues in Clinical Neuroscience 19: 93–107.

Guastella AJ, Howard AL, Dadds MR, et al. (2009) A randomised controlled trial of intranasal oxytocin as an adjunct to exposure therapy for social anxiety disorder. Psychoneuroendocrinology 34: 917–923.

Halverson T, Jarskog LF, Pedersen C, Penn D (2019) Effects of oxytocin on empathy, introspective accuracy and social symptoms in schizophrenia: a 12-week twice-daily randomised controlled trial. Schizophrenia Research 204: 178–182.

Kingsep P, Nathan P, Castle D (2003) Cognitive behavioural group treatment for social anxiety in schizophrenia. Schizophrenia Research 63: 121–129.

Liebowitz M (1987) Social phobia. Modern Problems of Pharmacopsychiatry 22: 141–173.

Lowengrub KM, Stryer R, Birger M, Iancu I (2015) Social anxiety disorder comorbid with schizophrenia: the importance of screening for this underrecognised and undertreated condition. Israeli Journal of Psychiatry and Related Sciences 52: 40–46.

McEnery C, Lim MH, Tremain H, et al. (2019) Prevalence rate of social anxiety disorder in individuals with a psychotic disorder: a systematic review and meta-analysis. Schizophrenia Research 208: 25–33.

Michail M, Birchwood M (2009) Social anxiety disorder in first-episode psychosis: incidence, phenomenology and relationship with paranoia. British Journal of Psychiatry 195: 234–241.

Pallanti S, Quercioli L, Hollander E (2004) Social anxiety in outpatients with schizophrenia: a relevant cause of disability. American Journal of Psychiatry 161: 53–58.

Romm KL, Rossberg JI, Berg AO, et al. (2011) Assessment of social anxiety in first episode psychosis using the Liebowitz Social Anxiety Scale as a self-report measure. European Psychiatry 26: 115–121.

Scheff TJ (1974) The labelling theory of mental illness. American Sociological Review 39: 444–452.

Wallace CJ, Nelson CJ, Liberman RP, et al. (1980) A review and critique of social skills training with schizophrenic patients. Schizophrenia Bulletin 6: 42–63.

CHAPTER 8

Schizophrenia and obsessive compulsive disorder

> **KEY POINTS**
>
> * Schizophrenia and OCD occur together much more commonly than would be expected by chance.
> * The reasons for this association include potential shared neurodevelopmental deviance and the induction of obsessive compulsive symptoms (OCS) by certain atypical antipsychotics.
> * People with schizophrenia and OCD often carry other psychiatric morbidities and experience a poor longitudinal illness course.
> * Treatment of people with schizophrenia and OCD usually targets psychotic symptoms first, and then addresses OCS.

The association between schizophrenia and OCD is particularly fascinating in that there are both phenomenological and aetiopathogenic aspects. Some phenomena manifested as part of OCD can be quite bizarre and could be confused with psychotic symptoms. There is also evidence that some people with OCD go on to develop schizophrenia, whilst others manifest a disorder in which both OCD and schizophrenia symptoms are present: this is sometimes referred to as 'schizo-obsessive' disorder. Finally, a number of antipsychotic medications—notably clozapine—can exacerbate or even induce OCD symptoms in people with schizophrenia. Cheng et al. (2019) suggest five possible sequences for the association between schizophrenia and OCD, summarized in Box 8.1.

How common is OCD in people with schizophrenia?

In the 1950s, Stengel recognized that people with schizophrenia are at increased risk of comorbid OCD, and his student Rosen (1957) duly reported a rate of OCD of 3.5% in a group of 848 people with schizophrenia. Those were the days when OCD was diagnosed very conservatively, and thus the reported rate was much higher than the general population rate. Subsequent studies have adopted more stringent methodology and larger samples, including non-clinical sampling frames. For example, using data from the US Epidemiological Catchment Area (ECA) study, Boyd and colleagues (1984) reported an Odds Ratio (OR) of 12.5 for OCD risk amongst people with schizophrenia, compared to the general population. Buckley et al. (2009) found 36 studies from a range of different settings

Box 8.1 Sequences of association of OCD and schizophrenia

* OCD occurring prior to schizophrenia
* OCD as part of a schizophrenia 'at risk' mental state
* OCD and schizophrenia onset at the same time
* OCD manifesting after the schizophrenia diagnosis
* OCD manifesting in a person with schizophrenia in the context of treatment with antipsychotic medication

(inpatient, day programme, community) and encompassing early episode and chronic schizophrenia samples: all bar one reported rates of OCD higher than those expected in the general population (range 0–32%). Higher rates tended to reflect the application of less stringent criteria for OCD in more recent editions of the DSM. Some studies avoided the diagnostic problem by simply reporting rates of OCS: here rates ranged from 10% to 60%.

Swets and colleagues (2014) performed a meta-analysis and meta-regression of 43 studies encompassing 3,978 individuals with schizophrenia and estimated a mean prevalence of OCD of 12.3%; for OCS the mean rate was 30.7%.

In terms of illness stage, features of OCD have been reported both in early and later stage schizophrenia. It is tempting to suggest that OCD is more common in people later on in the course of schizophrenia, but any such findings are highly inconsistent and in any event would be confounded by use of clozapine, which is mostly reserved for treatment-resistant schizophrenia and which has a strong signal for the induction of OCS. An excess of OCD has been shown in people at putative high risk for schizophrenia (DeVylder et al. 2012) as well as in the schizophrenia prodrome. Associations with comorbid OCD in schizophrenia are shown in Box 8.2.

How common is schizophrenia in people with OCD?

Whilst an excess of OCD in people with established schizophrenia has been widely reported, the issue of people who are initially diagnosed with OCD later manifesting schizophrenia has been less studied. The tracking of this sequence has important implications for our understanding of the pathophysiological under-pinnings of the association between the two disorders. Longitudinal studies from Sweden (Cederlöf et al. 2015) and Denmark (Meier et al. 2014) have reported increased rates of schizophrenia in people diagnosed with OCD: 2.7-fold in the former and 6.9 (incidence ratio) in the latter study. Most recently, in a popula-tion cohort study from Taiwan, Cheng et al. (2019) found that the risk of later

---

Box 8.2 Features associated with schizophrenia in which OCD is comorbid

- Early onset of psychotic illness
- Motor tics
- Body dysmorphic disorder
- Depression
- Suicidality
- Cognitive dysfunction (notably executive function)
- Poor social functionality
- High overall disability
- High hospitalization rates
- Exposure to atypical antipsychotics, notably clozapine

Source: Data from Buckley, P., Miller, B.J., Lehrer, D.S., Castle, D.J. (2009) Psychiatric comorbidities and schizophrenia. *Schizophrenia Bulletin*, 35: 383–402; Poyurovsky, M., Kriss, V., Weisman, G., et al. (2005) Familial aggregation of schizophrenia-spectrum disorders and obsessive-compulsive associated disorders in schizophrenia probands with and without schizophrenia. *American Journal of Medical Genetics B Neuropsychiatric Genetics*, 133: 31–36; Hadi, E., Greenberg, Y., Sirota, P. (2012) Obsessive-compulsive symptoms in schizophrenia: prevalence, clinical features and treatment: a literature review. *The World Journal of Biological Psychiatry*, 13: 2–13.

---

schizophrenia in people initially diagnosed with OCD (n=2,009) was 876.2 per 100,000 person years, whilst the risk in a non-OCD control sample (n=8,036: matched for age, sex, level of urbanization and income) was 28.7 per 100,000 person years. This represents an increased hazard in the OCD group of 30.2 (95% CI 17.9–51.2). Being male, having an OCD onset before age 20, comorbid autism spectrum disorder, and the prescription of antipsychotic medication were associated with a schizophrenia diagnosis. These associations suggest a profile of early onset, male preponderant neurodevelopmental deviance which increases risk for both schizophrenia and OCD and encompasses autism risk: this theory is expostulated in more detail below.

Why do schizophrenia and OCD occur together more often than by chance?

There are a number of theories as to why schizophrenia and OCD show such strong co-aggregation. Studies seeking a genetic explanation include that of Poyurovsky et al. (2005), which found an excess of both schizophrenia and OCD in the family members (n = 182) of probands with schizophrenia and OCD (n = 57) compared to those with schizophrenia alone (n = 60). These findings suggest some shared genetic predisposition to schizophrenia and OCD. Some commentators propose that there is a relatively discrete 'schizo-obsessive' subtype of schizophrenia, but one could equally argue for it being a subtype of OCD. Indeed, a neurodevelopmental subtype of OCD has long been hypothesized (e.g. Blanes and McGuire 1997): many features are shared with the putative neurodevelopmental subtype of schizophrenia (Murray et al. 1992): see Box 8.3.

There is a high degree of overlap between psychiatric disorders in general in terms of predisposing genes (see Chapter 1). Costas et al. (2016) explored the polygenic risk profiles of 370 individuals with OCD and 443 controls and compared them to an existing schizophrenia database. The polygenic risk model for schizophrenia was strongly associated with OCD, but was even stronger when the major histocompatibility complex region (one of the most robust genetic associations with schizophrenia) was removed from the modelling. These findings suggest overlap of genetic predisposition to schizophrenia and OCD, but also important differences.

Attempts at exploring the neurobiology of schizo-obsessive disorder have focused on neurocognitive domains that may be shared or differ across schizophrenia and schizo-obsessive disorder. Sahoo et al. (2018) compared 40 patients with schizophrenia and OCD with a matched sample of 39 people with schizophrenia alone. The comorbid group was more impaired on tests of processing speed, verbal fluency, cognitive flexibility and executive function. Neuroimaging studies have also been pursued. For example, Wang et al. (2019) compared resting state functional connectivity (rsFC) of the default mode network (DMN) in 22 people with schizo-obsessive disorder, 20 with schizophrenia alone, 22 with OCD and 22 healthy controls. The schizo-obsessive group showed highest rsFC strength within subregions of the DMN and lowest strength between the DMN and the salience network, suggesting a particular pattern of brain functional disorganization in these individuals.

Another approach to understanding the overlap between schizophrenia and OCD has been looking at neurochemical similarities and differences between the disorders. We tend to think of schizophrenia as essentially a disorder of

---

Box 8.3 Shared features of putative neurodevelopmental subtypes of OCD and schizophrenia

- Early illness onset
- Male sex
- Poor premorbid social adjustment
- Poor premorbid academic achievement
- Motor tics (OCD only)
- Neurological soft signs
- Poor longitudinal course

Source: Data from Blanes, T., McGuire, P. (1997) Heterogeneity within obsessive-compulsive disorder: evidence for primary and neurodevelopmental subtypes. In: Keshavan MS, Murray RM (eds) *Neurodevelopment and Adult Psychopathology*. Cambridge: Cambridge University Press, pp. 206–212; Murray, R.M., O'Callaghan, E., Castle, D.J., Lewis, S.W. (1992) A neurodevelopmental approach to the classification of schizophrenia. *Schizophrenia Bulletin*, 18: 319–332.

dopamine balance in the brain and of OCD as a disorder in which serotoninergic pathways are perturbed. But of course this is far too simplistic, and serotonergic and glutamatergic mechanisms are known to be operating in schizophrenia, whilst dopaminergic and glutamatergic circuitry have been strongly implicated in OCD. Heuristically, atypical antipsychotics (bar sulpride and amisulpride) have important serotonergic activity (notably blockade of serotonin 5HT2a receptors), and it is these agents that can exacerbate or cause de novo OCS/OCD in people with schizophrenia. The converse is that often antipsychotic medications can benefit people with OCD who do not respond simply to serotonin reuptake inhibitor antidepressants (Castle et al. 2015).

How do we differentiate the features of schizophrenia from OCD?

The differentiation of obsessive compulsive from psychotic symptoms is usually fairly straightforward. *Obsessions* are intrusive thoughts, recognized as the person's own and causing distress that is alleviated (at least to some extent, in the short term) by ritualized acts or thoughts. The obsessions are usually 'understandable' at some level: for example, that the toaster has been left on and might burn the house down. And the sufferer usually has at least partial insight in that they see their thoughts as excessive or even 'silly' and try to resist the urge to perform the rituals. In contrast, *delusions* are fixed false beliefs which may be bizarre and clearly outside what might be considered normal human experience. Unlike obsessional ruminations, psychotic hallucinations are heard through the ears and have all the features of a true experiential phenomenon.

But in many cases these distinctions become blurred. Some ruminations in people with OCD have a quite unusual character and the content can become 'believed' with psychotic tenacity by the individual. For example, a patient held a fixed belief that they could only move through doors with their head held at a certain angle and had to think a certain specific thought as they did so. They also did not have the 'usual' OCD-related belief that if they did not perform the ritual in this way some harm might befall another person; in this case their belief about what might ensue was much more 'mystical'—even grandiose—and ill-formulated, such that the world would suffer some catastrophe. Such beliefs verge on the psychotic and can be mistaken for psychotic symptoms.

Conversely, a patient with schizophrenia who had a clear persecutory delusional belief system, including the belief that she was being spied on and that there were cameras throughout the hospital ward, was commenced on clozapine. On the ward she was noted to be highly distressed and checking electrical fittings and light features. Initially it was thought that she was acting on her delusions, but when closely questioned it became clear that her psychotic symptoms had settled and her checking behaviours were driven by intervening obsessional beliefs

> **Box 8.4** Differentiating obsessive compulsive from psychotic symptoms
>
> * Thematic content of obsessions representative of OCD (e.g. cleanliness, orderliness)
> * Perceived consequence of not performing rituals relate to common OCD themes (e.g. harm befalling another person)
> * Usually have at least partial insight
> * Rituals are performed to alleviate anxiety associated with the compulsions, and are usually to some extent resisted
> * Form of thought may be circumstantial/overinclusive in OCD but usually does not decompensate as severely (e.g. tangentiality, derailment) as in schizophrenia
> * Negative symptoms are not usually a feature of OCD

related to the fear that if she did not check, the ward might burn down. These symptoms responded well to the addition of a serotonin reuptake inhibitor to her clozapine.

In cases where there is a blurring of features between OCD and psychotic symptoms that are part of a psychotic process illness, a number of questions can be applied, as outlined in Box 8.4. One particular diagnostic complexity is seen in early onset severe OCD with primary obsessional slowness: this can be very difficult to disentangle from a psychotic process illness, but usually the reason for the slowness is able to be articulated by the person with OCD (e.g. due to the 'need' to perform mental rituals).

Another consideration is that some people have a putative subtype of schizophrenia with overlapping obsessive compulsive phenomena: so-called schizo-obsessive disorder. Here one might see a mix of features, including obsessions and compulsions as well as bizarre delusions and true hallucinations, in association with negative symptoms and formal thought disorder. The possible aetiopathogenesis of this disorder is outlined above. The treatment approach is usually pragmatically based on treating the ameliorable psychotic features first, and then addressing residual obsessive compulsive phenomena: this is explained further below.

How do we treat OCD symptoms in people with schizophrenia?

In psychiatry generally we tend to adopt a hierarchical approach to diagnosis and treatment. In the setting of comorbid schizophrenia and OCD, this means that we usually treat the schizophrenia symptoms first, and then address the OCD symptoms. Of course exceptions can be made, for example if the OCD symptoms are highly distressing and disabling and the psychotic symptoms less prominent. What is vital is that each set of symptoms is monitored and targeted, and also that the impact of each set of symptoms is assessed in an ongoing manner.

The treatment of schizophrenia itself is beyond the scope of this book, and the reader is referred to other books in this series (notably Castle and Buckley 2015) and appropriate treatment guidelines. For the purposes of this chapter, it must be noted that some antipsychotics can exacerbate OCS or even cause them to manifest for the first time. As outlined above, this has been described mostly with those 'atypical' antipsychotics that have affinity for the serotonin 5HT2a receptor, implicating serotonergic pathways, albeit the precise mechanisms are not fully understood and dopaminergic and glutamatergic mechanisms are also likely to play a role (Laroche and Gaillard 2016).

In some cases, consideration might be given to changing the antipsychotic to an agent with lower risk of OCS (e.g. typical antipsychotics, amisulpride). Having said this, if the chosen antipsychotic is otherwise effective and well tolerated, the evolution of OCS should not necessarily predicate withdrawal of the implicated agent; this is particularly the case with clozapine as it is often the most effective antipsychotic in people 'resistant' to other antipsychotics. Usually the OCS can be managed with the addition of targeted psychological therapy in conjunction with a serotonergic reuptake inhibitor (SRI) antidepressant. This would certainly be a sensible approach if the individual also had a depressive disorder. For a detailed account of antidepressant use in schizophrenia the reader is referred to Chapter 10.

Care should be taken regarding certain pharmacokinetic interactions with antidepressants, notably fluvoxamine and clozapine (each can raise the serum levels of the other): citalopram, escitalopram and sertraline are suggested as the SRIs least likely to cause troublesome interactions. With any anti-obsessional drug, cumulative side effects can be problematic: for example, sexual dysfunction can occur with antipsychotics and with SRIs. There is also some evidence that in some people with schizophrenia, antidepressants can exacerbate psychotic symptoms or cause aggressive behaviours (Poyurovsky et al. 2004). An alternative to SRIs is the partial dopamine agonist aripiprazole (Laroche and Gaillard 2016).

Poyurovsky et al. (2004) suggested a step-wise approach to the medication management of people with schizophrenia and comorbid OCD or schizo-obsessive disorder, as outlined in Box 8.5. Of course each step needs to be accompanied by a full discussion with the patient as well as close monitoring for efficacy and side effects. The evidence base becomes scarcer the further along the algorithm. Note also the issues with clozapine potentially worsening the OCS, but some clinical data suggest efficacy in some people with schizo-obsessive disorder.

Conclusions

OCD occurs more often than chance in people with schizophrenia, and vice versa. The reasons for this are not fully understood, but a conceptualization that neurodevelopmental processes converge in the development of both

Box 8.5 Medication management of people with comorbid schizophrenia and OCD

* Atypical antipsychotic monotherapy
* If residual OCS, add an SSRI
* If ineffective, switch to a different SSRI
* If ineffective, switch antipsychotic to a typical agent
* If ineffective, try low-dose clozapine
* If ineffective, add an SSRI to clozapine
* If ineffective, try electroconvulsive therapy (ECT)

Adapted with permission from Poyurovsky, M., Weizman, A., Weizman, R. Obsessive-compulsive disorder and schizophrenia: Clinical characteristics and treatment. *CNS Drugs*, 18: 989–1010. Copyright © 2012, Springer Nature.

these symptom sets in some people (so-called schizo-obsessive disorder) has parsimony. Another pathway to people with schizophrenia developing OCD is through the action of certain antipsychotics, notably clozapine. Treatment is usually focused on the psychotic symptoms first, then targeting OCS with psychological therapy, usually in conjunction with SSRIs; sometimes other strategies are required to enhance functionality of the individual.

REFERENCES

Blanes T, McGuire P (1997) Heterogeneity within obsessive-compulsive disorder: evidence for primary and neurodevelopmental subtypes. In: Keshavan MS, Murray RM (eds) Neurodevelopment and Adult Psychopathology. Cambridge: Cambridge University Press, pp. 206–212.

Buckley P, Miller BJ, Lehrer DS, Castle DJ (2009) Psychiatric comorbidities and schizophrenia. Schizophrenia Bulletin 35: 383–402.

Castle DJ, Rossell S, Bosanac P (2015) Treating OCD: what to do when first line therapies fail. Australasian Psychiatry 23: 350–353.

Cederlöf M, Lichtenstein P, Larsson H, et al. (2015) Obsessive-compulsive disorder, psychosis, and bipolarity: a longitudinal cohort and multigenerational family study. Schizophrenia Bulletin 41: 1076–1083.

Cheng Y-F, Chen VCH, Yang YH, et al. (2019) Risk of schizophrenia among people with obsessive-compulsive disorder: a nationwide population-based cohort study. Schizophrenia Research 209: 58–63.

Costas J, Carrera N, Alonso P, et al. (2016) Exon-focussed genome-wide association study of obsessive-compulsive disorder and shared polygenic risk with schizophrenia. Translational Psychiatry 6: e768.

DeVylder JE, Oh AJ, Ben-David S, et al. (2012) Obsessive compulsive symptoms in individuals at clinical risk for psychosis: association with depressive symptoms and suicidal ideation. Schizophrenia Research 140: 110–113.

Hadi E, Greenberg Y, Sirota P (2012) Obsessive-compulsive symptoms in schizophrenia: prevalence, clinical features and treatment: a literature review. The World Journal of Biological Psychiatry 13: 2–13.

Laroche DG, Gaillard A (2016) Induced obsessive compulsive symptoms (OCS) in schizophrenia patients with atypical 2 antipsychotics (AAPs): review and hypotheses. Psychiatry Research 246: 119–128.

Meier SM, Petersen L, Pedersen MG, et al. (2014) Obsessive-compulsive disorder as a risk factor for schizophrenia: a nationwide study. JAMA Psychiatry 71: 1215–1221.

Murray RM, O'Callaghan E, Castle DJ, Lewis SW (1992) A neurodevelopmental approach to the classification of schizophrenia. Schizophrenia Bulletin 18: 319–332.

Poyurovsky M, Weizman A, Weizman R (2004) Obsessive-compulsive disorder and schizophrenia: clinical characteristics and treatment. CNS Drug 18: 989–1010.

Poyurovsky M, Kriss V, Weisman G, et al. (2005) Familial aggregation of schizophrenia-spectrum disorders and obsessive-compulsive associated disorders in schizophrenia probands with and without schizophrenia. American Journal of Medical Genetics B Neuropsychiatric Genetics 133: 31–36.

Poyurovsky M, Faragian S, Shabeta A, Kosov A (2008) Comparison of clinical characteristics, comorbidity and pharmacotherapy in adolescent schizophrenia patients with and without obsessive-compulsive disorder. Psychiatry Research 159: 133–139.

Rosen I (1957) The clinical significance of obsessions in schizophrenia. Journal of Mental Science 53: 773–785.

Sahoo S, Grover S, Nehra R (2018) Comparison of neurocognitive domains in patients with schizophrenia with and without comorbid obsessive-compulsive disorder. Schizophrenia Research 201: 151–158.

Swets M, Dekker J, van Emmerik-van Oortmerssen K, et al. (2014) The obsessive-compulsive spectrum in schizophrenia, a meta-analysis and meta-regression exploring prevalence rates. Schizophrenia Research 152: 458–468.

Wang Y-M, Zou L-Q, Xie W-L, et al. (2019) Altered functional connectivity of the default mode network in patients with schizo-obsessive comorbidity: a comparison between schizophrenia and obsessive-compulsive disorder. Schizophrenia Bulletin 45: 199–210.

CHAPTER 9

Post-traumatic stress disorder and schizophrenia

KEY POINTS

- Schizophrenia and post-traumatic stress disorder (PTSD) occur together much more commonly than would be expected by chance.
- There is evidence that there are common aetiological antecedents to both psychosis and PTSD, including childhood trauma and other adverse experiences.
- Psychosis itself (persecutory delusions, malevolent voices, acts carried out in response to psychosis) can be traumatic and re-traumatizing for those with a significant past history.
- Coercive treatment can also compound the traumatic experience of psychosis: e.g. detention in hospital, physical restraint, locked wards.
- Comorbid PTSD significantly reduces the chance of a full recovery and remission.
- Attention should be paid to the long-term impact of trauma in schizophrenia, and in particular to the identification, and prevention, of factors that may increase PTSD.

Trauma and psychosis go hand in hand. Many traumatic experiences, such as childhood adversity, deprivation, and minority group status can be considered as aetiopathological events in the development of schizophrenia. Schizophrenia itself is traumatic in many aspects, including the experience of symptoms themselves, events that can occur in the context of acute behavioural disturbance, and treatment itself. Therefore it should be no surprise that PTSD symptoms occur more frequently than chance in people with schizophrenia. Furthermore, PTSD can significantly exacerbate poor outcomes and therefore represents a significant target for treatment.

Incidence and prevalence

PTSD is defined as the occurrence of symptoms of greater than one month duration, including re-experiencing distressing aspects of the trauma, hyper-arousal, avoidance of trauma reminders, sleep disturbances, and negative cognitions and mood, that typically develop after experiencing or witnessing an event or events that involve actual or threatened death or injury, of significant physical integrity to self or others (Association 2013) (see Box 9.1). There is growing evidence that

Box 9.1 Summary of salient features of PTSD

* Exposure to a significant traumatic event or series of events
* Intrusion symptoms:
  * Intrusive memories
  * Recurrent dreams
  * Dissociative reactions
  * Psychological distress in response to triggering cues
  * Physiological arousal in response to triggering cues
* Avoidance behaviours
* Negative alterations in cognitions and mood associated with the trauma
* Alterations in arousal and reactivity:
  * Irritable and angry outbursts
  * Recklessness
  * Hyper-vigilance
  * Exaggerated startle response
  * Poor concentration
  * Sleep disturbance

Source: Data from American Psychiatric Association, *Diagnostic and Statistical Manual of Mental Disorders*, 5th edition (DSM-5), 2013, American Psychiatric Association.

people with a severe mental illness are more vulnerable to PTSD due to increased risk of childhood and adulthood trauma and the experience of psychosis itself. Traumatic events themselves are highly prevalent in severe mental illness, with up to 90% of subjects reporting trauma (Lommen and Restifo 2009).

In cross-sectional studies, up to 30% of patients with schizophrenia meet diagnostic criteria for PTSD, albeit the aggregated risk estimates across studies are more in the order of 12% (see Chapter 2). An 18-month follow-up of first episode patients reported 31% developing PTSD, and substance abuse is a further risk association, such that nearly two-thirds of patients with schizophrenia and comorbid substance misuse have been reported to also meet criteria for PTSD (Grubaugh et al. 2011; Jackson et al. 2009; Seow et al. 2016).

Causation

Shared risk factors and mechanisms

Adverse events in childhood and early adulthood increase the risk of psychosis (see Box 9.2). Parental loss, bullying, and childhood abuse occur more frequently than chance in the lives of people with psychotic disorders. These traumatic events may be acting on an underlying (genomic or epigenetic) vulnerability, triggering psychosis. Indeed, one current mechanistic hypothesis centres on maternal

> **Box 9.2** Models of PTSD in schizophrenia
>
> • Trauma as a common risk factor: comorbid categorical diagnoses with shared antecedents
> • PTSD in response to psychosis as a traumatic event
> • Misclassification of symptoms

immune activation, whereby early pro-inflammatory insult (maternal stress, viral exposure, etc.) leads to a heighted inflammatory response when a second trigger occurs—the second trigger being an environmental challenge, including traumatic events. Immune activation, insufficient oxidative defence, and/or secondary glutamatergic and striatal dopaminergic changes are then secondary effects (Upthegrove and Khandaker 2019). It is parsimonious that those who are more vulnerable to psychosis may also be more likely to experience early trauma (Seow et al. 2016). Thus, the same events that can predispose to schizophrenia could lead to the development of PTSD in addition to psychosis.

PTSD in response to psychosis

A psychotic episode might itself be viewed as a life event sufficiently traumatic to trigger PTSD symptoms. There is clear evidence that psychosis can be extremely distressing and traumatic and may be valid as a PTSD triggering event. The experience of persecutory delusions held with conviction and in which the patient gathers more and more confirmatory evidence is often extremely traumatic and is perceived with conviction as a threat to self. Malevolent, complex, fully formed hallucinations threatening personal integrity or the threat to the very idea of self that occurs with passivity experiences can be sufficiently traumatic to initiate a process culminating in PTSD symptoms (Jackson et al. 2004). Psychological models of PTSD suggest that it is the *subjective* perception of threat that is more important than the *objective* assessment of threat; and it is an individual *appraisal* of the event and of sequelae and anticipated consequences that is the determinant of what is defined as a traumatic event. The experience and appraisal of positive symptoms of psychosis are key factors in relation to the traumatic experience of psychosis: for example, the powerfulness of persecutors and voices, helplessness of the individual, and conviction of threat (Freeman and Garety 2003; Jackson et al. 2004; Michail and Birchwood 2009).

Appraisal of the diagnosis of psychosis, hospitalization, and coercive treatment during first episode psychosis are also reported to predict PTSD (Jackson et al. 2004). The first admission to hospital can be the most distressing. Meyer et al. reported that 24% of PTSD symptoms following psychosis were related to recurrent intrusive experiences of hospitalization. There is also the prospect of re-traumatization, with higher rates of childhood trauma in those more likely to experience psychosis, and then traumatic psychotic symptoms and/or inpatient experiences compounding the impact of trauma in psychosis. In counterbalance, the events that may lead to a decision for hospital admission, for example acts of self-harm completed in response to command hallucinations or delusions of passivity or acting on bizarre delusional beliefs, may also be traumatic (Michail and Birchwood 2009) and individual risks and history need to be taken into account.

The relationship between the experience of coercive treatment of psychosis and PTSD may not be straight forward. Jackson et al. (2004) demonstrated, in a follow-up of first episode patients who experienced potentially traumatic events such as detention under The Mental Health Act, that hospital treatment per se was not as relevant as the subjective appraisal of the stressfulness of inpatient care together with individual coping style, in determining adverse psychological outcomes. Moreover, individuals more likely to 'seal over' experiences were less likely to report arousal and intrusions (Jackson et al. 2004). This is particularly relevant when considering working on insight and early warning signs, in that assessment of coping style may be as important as experiences of potentially traumatic events; subjective appraisals are key. However, in weighing up the balance of coercive treatment and risk management, clinicians should be fully aware of the potential for trauma, re-traumatization, and the impact this may have on longer-term outcomes.

Symptoms of PTSD 'misclassified' as psychosis

Despite the apparent distinction between categorical diagnoses such as schizophrenia and anxiety disorders, there are similarities at a symptom-specific level that should not be overlooked. It is possible that some of the high ratings of PTSD symptoms in psychosis are in fact related to undertreated or underrecognized positive symptoms, or indeed that both PTSD and positive symptoms are less distinguishable than first thought. As an example we can consider hallucinations and flashbacks. In traditional psychopathology, hallucinations are experienced as sense perceptions with all the vividness and fullness of real perceptions, without an objective source. Flashbacks are the re-experiencing of traumatic events with full emersion in sensory perception, often with dissociation and retained insight. The potential overlap is perhaps most evident with visual hallucinations occurring with retained insight, but auditory hallucinations and multisensory hallucinations can also be seen in schizophrenia patients who have a trauma history. In addition, hyper-vigilance, attention to potential threat, and external attributions are key in cognitive models of the development of paranoid delusions, yet are core features of PTSD. Alsawy et al. (2015) explored the specific psychotic symptoms associated with PTSD; arousal and flashbacks (re-living) experiences were more associated with paranoia than hallucinations, whereas multiple traumas were associated with both paranoia and hallucinations (Alsawy et al. 2015).

In addition, negative symptoms such as emotional blunting and social withdrawal may be difficult to distinguish from trauma-related avoidance. Thorough exploration of the subjective experience of emotions and reason behind withdrawal is needed. Secondary negative symptoms, such as undertreated paranoid ideation or anhedonia related to depression, need careful consideration (Muenzenmaier et al. 2005).

Whilst it is clear that PTSD and schizophrenia have distinguishable trajectories in their respective categorical diagnoses, even when present in comorbidity, PTSD can be reliably assessed in people with schizophrenia and should not be overlooked (Buckley et al. 2009). The concept of misclassification of 'true' PTSD and 'true' schizophrenia is possibly unhelpful: multiple traumas and childhood adversities increase the risk of psychosis, and complex psychopathology is likely to follow complex traumatic experiences.

Management of PTSD in people with schizophrenia

A diagnosis of PTSD in a person with a psychotic disorder predicts more severe mental health outcomes, greater use of health and psychiatric services, lower satisfaction with services, increased suicidal ideation and acts, and poorer life satisfaction. Unrecognized PTSD may also lead to increased risk of re-traumatization and ineffective treatment if PTSD symptoms are interpreted simply as being part of the psychotic disorder (see above). It is therefore essential that PTSD is recognized *and* effectively treated in order to achieve maximum recovery potentials with any given patient, and there is growing evidence that PTSD can be treated in this population (Jackson et al. 2009; Michail and Birchwood 2009). Box 9.3 summarizes treatment approaches.

Pharmacological treatment

We are aware of no published trials that have been specifically designed to investigate effectiveness of pharmacotherapy for PTSD in schizophrenia (Braga et al. 2013). Evidence that does exist thus needs to be gleaned from trials of PTSD in people without comorbid schizophrenia. As outlined in other chapters of this book, this suggests limited evidence to warrant individual patient trials with SSRIs, with care to avoid ineffective polypharmacy. Taking evidence from the

---

Box 9.3 Treatment of PTSD in schizophrenia

- Very little conclusive evidence exists for pharmacological or psychological interventions
- Antidepressant medication and EMDR are likely to be safe in schizophrenia
- Prolonged exposure could be re-traumatizing and great care needs to be exercised in using this paradigm in people with schizophrenia
- Service structures and provision of mental health care should recognize the prevalence of PTSD in schizophrenia and be better designed to prevent traumatic pathways to care and re-traumatization

EMDR, Eye movement desensitization and reprocessing.

pharmacological management of PTSD without schizophrenia, evidence exists to favour the SSRIs sertraline and paroxetine in those over the age of 18 (Kelmendi et al. 2016). Venlafaxine may also be of some benefit (National Institute for Health and Care Excellence (NICE) 2018). Benzodiazepines should generally be avoided. Medications acting on GABAergic pathways, such as gabapentin and pregabalin, have as yet uncertain longer-term dependence potential and should be used with due caution, if at all, in this context (Evoy et al. 2017). Novel therapies in development for the treatment of PTSD include cannabinoids which are also being considered for the adjunctive treatment of positive and negative symptoms of psychosis (Ney et al. 2019), as well as ketamine (DePierro et al. 2019); however, there is insufficient evidence to speculate on their effectiveness in treatment of trauma in schizophrenia.

Psychological treatment

The gold-standard psychological treatment for PTSD is exposure therapy, where patients are encouraged to gradually confront reminders of their trauma, enabling them to learn to regulate their fear of the no-longer threatening situation. This may be challenging or indeed damaging in schizophrenia, whereby experiences are complex, may be related to psychopathology, or may be difficult to recreate (e.g. detention, coercive hospital admission). A recent Cochrane review summarized evidence for psychological treatment of PTSD in patients with severe mental illness, defined as a non-organic psychosis with significant impairment and a treatment duration of over two years. In this review, Sin et al. (2017) identified four trials, with a total n= 300, investigating (i) trauma-focused cognitive behavioural therapy (TF-CBT) and (ii) eye movement desensitization and reprocessing (EMDR), both evaluated compared to each other and usual care/waiting list. Individual studies were small, had short follow-up, and were of low to very low quality evidence. One larger trial of EMDR offered evidence of safety and effect sizes for EMDR comparably to prolonged exposure therapy in reducing symptoms. Compared to usual care/waiting list, no difference was found for TF-CBT on PTSD symptoms, while one trial reported a positive effect of EMDR on PTSD symptoms (n=83, standardized mean difference (SMD) −12.31). Compared to each other, there was no difference on outcomes. Sin et al. (2017) concluded that TF-CBT and EMDR have a very limited and inconclusive evidence of effectiveness on PTSD in severe mental illness.

Given the prominence of PTSD in early psychosis, psychological interventions have also focused on treatment in these earlier stages, although without a sufficient body of work for definitive guidance to be drawn. NICE guidelines in the UK recommend that early intervention services should monitor and assess for PTSD; thus there is need for evidence-based treatments in early phases to match this monitoring (NICE 2017). One case series has been published and Valiante-Gomez et al. plan a phase II rater blind randomized controlled trial of EMDR with 80 FEP patients with a history of trauma, but outcomes are yet to be reported (Valiente-Gómez et al. 2020; Ward-Brown et al. 2018).

Conclusions

Recognizing the potential for PTSD and traumatization through the experience of psychosis has potentially significant implications for the planning of treatment services and their structure. Prevention of trauma and re-traumatization should have great emphasis in the planning and development of services for people with severe mental illness. Increased focus on engagement, early intervention, social recovery, and avoidance of coercive treatment would appear a sensible approach and are the cornerstone of specialist psychosis services where they exist. On the other hand, positive symptoms can be potentially equally traumatic and there is a careful balance that needs to be drawn, with the individual case and specific risk factors in mind (Marwaha et al. 2016). It is indeed unfortunate that poorly funded mental health services, or those well funded but lacking sufficient community-based interventions, may not be able to offer alternatives to hospital-based care even when this is warranted, and which would reduce risks and improve outcomes.

REFERENCES

Alsawy S, Wood L, Taylor P, Morrison A (2015) Psychotic experiences and PTSD: exploring associations in a population survey. Psychological Medicine 45: 2849–2859.

American Psychiatric Association (2013) Diagnostic and Statistical Manual of Mental Disorders (DSM-5). Washington, DC: American Psychiatric Association.

Braga RJ, Reynolds GP, Siris SG (2013) Anxiety comorbidity in schizophrenia. Psychiatry Research 210: 1–7.

Buckley PF, Miller BJ, Lehrer DS, Castle DJ (2009) Psychiatric comorbidities and schizophrenia. Schizophrenia Bulletin 35: 383–402.

Depierro J, Lepow L, Feder A, Yehuda R (2019) Translating molecular and neuroendocrine findings in PTSD and resilience to novel therapies. Biological Psychiatry 86: 454–463.

Evoy KE, Morrison MD, Saklad SR (2017) Abuse and misuse of pregabalin and gabapentin. Drugs 77: 403–426.

Freeman D, Garety PA (2003) Connecting neurosis and psychosis: the direct influence of emotion on delusions and hallucinations. Behaviour Research and Therapy 41: 923–947.

Grubaugh AL, Zinzow HM, Paul L, Egede LE, Frueh BC (2011) Trauma exposure and posttraumatic stress disorder in adults with severe mental illness: a critical review. Clinical Psychology Review 31: 883–899.

Jackson C, Knott C, Skeate A, Birchwood M (2004) The trauma of first episode psychosis: the role of cognitive mediation. Australian and New Zealand Journal of Psychiatry 38: 327–333.

Jackson C, Trower P, Reid I, et al. (2009) Improving psychological adjustment following a first episode of psychosis: a randomised controlled trial of cognitive therapy to reduce post psychotic trauma symptoms. Behaviour Research and Therapy 47: 454–462.

Kelmendi B, Adams TG, Yarnell S, Southwick S, Abdallah CG, Krystal JH (2016) PTSD: from neurobiology to pharmacological treatments. European Journal of Psychotraumatology 7: 31858.

Lommen MJ, Restifo K (2009) Trauma and posttraumatic stress disorder (PTSD) in patients with schizophrenia or schizoaffective disorder. Community Mental Health Journal 45: 485.

Marwaha S, Thompson A, Upthegrove R, Broome MR (2016) Fifteen years on—early intervention for a new generation. British Journal of Psychiatry 209: 186–188.

Michail M, Birchwood M (2009) Social anxiety disorder in first-episode psychosis: incidence, phenomenology and relationship with paranoia. British Journal of Psychiatry 195: 234–241.

Muenzenmaier K, Jamison A, Battaglia J, Opler LA (2005) Comorbid posttraumatic stress disorder and schizophrenia. Psychiatric Annals 35: 50.

Ney L, Matthews A, Bruno R, Felmingham K (2019) Cannabinoid interventions for PTSD: where to next? Progress in Neuro-Psychopharmacology and Biological Psychiatry 93: 124–140.

NICE (2018). Post-Traumatic Stress Disorder. Guideline NG 116. London: NICE.

Seow LSE, Ong C, Mahesh MV, et al. (2016) A systematic review on comorbid post-traumatic stress disorder in schizophrenia. Schizophrenia Research 176: 441–451.

Upthegrove R, Khandaker GM (2019) Cytokines, oxidative stress and cellular markers of inflammation in schizophrenia.

Valiente-Gómez A, Pujol N, Moreno-Alcázar A, et al. (2020) A multicenter phase II RCT to compare the effectiveness of EMDR versus TAU in patients with a first-episode psychosis and psychological trauma: a protocol design. Frontiers in Psychiatry 10: 1023.

Ward-Brown J, Keane D, Bhutani G, Malkin D, Sellwood B, Varese F (2018) TF-CBT and EMDR for young people with trauma and first episode psychosis (using a phasic treatment approach): two early intervention service case studies. The Cognitive Behaviour Therapist 11: e17.

Depression and schizophrenia

KEY POINTS

* Comorbid depression is frequent, particularly in early stages of schizophrenia.
* Comorbid depression is a poor prognostic indicator for functional recovery, quality of life and suicide.
* Negative symptoms may be secondary to depression.
* SSRIs are generally safe to use for depression in the context of schizophrenia and are likely to be effective.
* Less evidence exists for CBTp and other psychosocial treatments, but those focused on hopelessness and reducing social isolation should be considered.

For many years the 'Kraepelinian dichotomy' that separated bipolar disorder and schizophrenia has been challenged. The presence of mood symptoms, and in particular depressive symptoms, is common in schizophrenia, as is the presence of first rank positive symptoms in bipolar disorder. Diagnostic fluidity is a key component in early stages of schizophrenia such as FEP, and depressive episodes are particularly common in this early phase of illness. Depression in the early stage may have long-term impacts in terms of suicidal behaviour and also functional outcome and relapse risk. However, existing treatments for depression do work in schizophrenia. Monitoring for significant mood symptoms in FEP and also later in the course of schizophrenia is essential in order to develop appropriate treatment plans.

Prevalence and importance of depression

Depression as a discrete syndrome is relatively common in schizophrenia, with a prevalence in cross-sectional studies of around 25–30% (Conley et al. 2007; Hafner et al. 2005); longitudinal studies show rates of over 50%. Prevalence figures for depressive features are higher still. In earlier phases of illnesses, such as the UHR phase, 40% of patients may meet criteria for a syndromal diagnosis of depression and this may be up to 80% of FEP patients in longitudinal studies. Depression in FEP thus occurs in prodromal, acute, and post-psychotic phases and classical post-psychotic depression rarely occurs unheralded by previous episodes (Upthegrove et al. 2010; Yung et al. 2006). See Box 10.1.

When depression is comorbid to any health disorder, there is a negative impact on the overall illness burden, and this is also the case in schizophrenia. Previously

Box 10.1 Prevalence of depressive episodes and depressive symptoms in schizophrenia

- In cross-sectional studies up to 40% of patients with schizophrenia are depressed
- Highest rates are seen early in the course of illness
- Longitudinally, the majority of patients with schizophrenia experience a depressive episode of at least moderate severity
- Post-psychotic depression is often preceded by depression in the prodrome or acute phases, and rarely arises 'de novo'

it has been proposed that depression in early psychosis may represent an individual patient's trajectory leaning towards a more affective rather than non-affective psychosis, and hence a better outcome. However, it is now fairly clear that depression has largely negative consequences in schizophrenia. Depression in schizophrenia is associated with more frequent psychotic episodes (Buckley et al. 2009), longer duration of illness, substance abuse, poor quality of life, and suicide. Depression during and after FEP is the most significant risk factor for suicidal behaviour; 35 out of every 100 patients with FEP may have attempted suicide, and completed suicide is most common in these early years of illness (Dutta et al. 2011; Upthegrove et al. 2010). In a systematic review and meta-analysis, depression after FEP was shown to have a longer-term impact on the likelihood of suicidal behaviour, lasting up to 7 years (McGinty et al. 2017). Depression in schizophrenia also has impacts on systems outside of the individual and on the healthcare burden, with greater use of mental health services and the criminal justice system (Conley et al. 2007). See Box 10.2.

Causation

That depression is common in schizophrenia should not come as a surprise, given the impact, stigma, and loss that may accompany any severe illness. There is also

Box 10.2 Importance of depressive episodes and depressive symptoms in schizophrenia

- Despite previous considerations, depression comorbidity is now known to be a poor prognostic indicator in schizophrenia
- Depression is significantly associated with increased risk of suicidal behaviour
- Depression is related to poorer recovery and reduced quality of life
- Patients with schizophrenia and depression are more likely to experience coercive forms of treatment

some limited biological evidence suggesting putative common aetiological pathways for symptoms of depression and positive psychotic symptoms, including systematic whole-genome linkage studies which have implicated chromosomal regions in common (International Schizophrenia Consortium 2009); brain imaging studies with similarities in both structural grey and white matter (Cui et al. 2011); and functional abnormalities in some key areas including the hippocampus, and prefrontal and frontal regions (Busatto 2013; Palaniyappan et al. 2019). Current biological models indicate commonality in pro-inflammatory cytokines and other innate immune markers; these are elevated in both depression and schizophrenia, and more so in those patients when both disorders occur together (Khandaker et al. 2014; Noto et al. 2015; Upthegrove et al. 2014). Furthermore, a number of studies have found that depression and anxiety tend to increase before the onset of a psychotic relapse, suggesting that affective dysfunction, rather than simply being a comorbidity, may be causally related to psychosis (Hall 2017).

There have been a number of quantitative and qualitative studies of depression in FEP and schizophrenia that have identified significant associations with the experience of positive symptoms, including powerful perceived persecutors, and commanding and authoritative hallucinations. Freeman and Garety have developed considerable evidence about powerfulness of persecutory beliefs and the adoption of safety behaviours (e.g. avoidance) that are important in emotional dysfunction in psychosis (Freeman and Garety 2003; Garety et al. 2001). It has also been demonstrated that depression emerging after psychosis is strongly associated with the loss of role and social status and internalized shame related to the experience and diagnosis of psychosis. Negative self-appraisals are common cognitive distortions also seen in non-psychotic depression, and intimately linked to past experience and the generation and perpetuation of depressive cognitions; similar psychological processes leading to depression in psychosis should be considered (Upthegrove et al. 2017).

In summary, models of depression in schizophrenia indicate that shared biological pathways, psychological response to the event of psychosis itself, and shared common factors, for example trauma, may all be indicated. Indeed, these are not mutually exclusive (see Chapter 3).

Recognition

The phenomenological symptoms of depression in schizophrenia are broadly similar to those found in major depressive disorder. However, some evidence suggests that negative cognitive appraisals of shame and loss are more prominent in post-psychotic depression as compared with major depressive disorder in other contexts (Häfner 2005; Sandhu et al. 2013). Also, acute phases of psychosis depression may be related to the experience of perceived threat from powerful persecutors and/or malevolent hallucinations (Birchwood et al. 2005; Garety et al. 2001).

Box 10.3 Assessment of depression in schizophrenia

* Carefully assess for negative symptoms and EPSE
* Consider completing a specific rating scale, e.g. the CDS
* Have particular focus on hopelessness and suicidal thinking
* Monitor functional recovery, and consider depression in all who do not fully recover

EPSE, Extrapyramidal side effects.

There are a number of features common to both depression and negative symptoms of psychosis, such as social withdrawal, anhedonia and anergia (Krynicki et al. 2018). There may be some distinction between consummatory anhedonia and anticipatory anhedonia. Depression can be masked or misinterpreted as negative symptoms, with the distinction between primary negative symptoms and secondary (to depression, antipsychotic medication, enduring positive symptoms) needing careful examination. Hopelessness and suicidality may be significant distinctions.

The CDS (Addington et al. 1993) is a brief, useful assessment schedule specifically developed for use in people with schizophrenia. It encompasses nine items covering:

* depressed mood
* hopelessness
* self-depreciation
* guilty ideas of reference
* pathological guilt
* morning depression
* early wakening
* suicidal thinking
* observed depression.

Management

Pharmacological interventions

There has been some recent strengthening of evidence for the pharmacological treatment of depression in schizophrenia. Updated British Association for Psychopharmacology (BAP) guidelines conclude that although large-scale definitive trials are still needed, enough evidence of the effectiveness and safety of co-prescribing antidepressants with antipsychotics means that cautious individual patient trials are warranted (Barnes et al. 2019). Helfer and colleagues (2016) conducted a meta-analysis of studies addressing the safety and efficacy of anti-depressants added to antipsychotic medication in the treatment of depression in people with schizophrenia. Adding an antidepressant to antipsychotic medication was found to be more efficacious than placebo or no intervention for the control of depressive symptoms, with an SMD across studies of –0.25 (95% CI –0.38 to –0.12) (see Figure 10.1). When patients had more severe depression, the effect sizes were higher. It may be concluded that co-prescribing an antipsychotic medication and an antidepressant is a combination that may produce some beneficial effects (Gregory et al. 2017; Helfer et al. 2016).

Polypharmacy is not without potential risks in people with severe mental illness, and concomitant use of antidepressants with antipsychotic medication may lead to increased cardiac effects and overall side effect burden. Having said this, Tiihonen and colleagues reviewed the co-prescribing of antidepressants with antipsychotic medication in a large population cohort and found that antidepressant use was not associated with a higher risk for mortality, yet was significantly associated with a decreased risk of completed suicide (Tiihonen et al. 2012).

Other considerations to make are the choice of antipsychotic and dose pre-scribed. There is some limited evidence that second generation antipsychotics (SGAs) may be less associated with depression than first generation agents (FGAs), possibly a legacy of depressive symptoms in schizophrenia being understood as the result of a depressogenic side effect of FGAs (Häfner 2005). Emsley et al. (2003) demonstrated a significant improvement in depression with quetiapine as compared to haloperidol. Both NICE and BAP guidance outline a clear benefit for the use of an SGA for augmentation of antidepressant medication for treatment-resistant depression (Barnes et al. 2019; Cleare et al. 2015). Leucht et al. reported that clozapine, quetiapine, olanzapine and aripiprazole may have a higher indi-vidual effect on depression in schizophrenia, albeit the clinical significance of the effect size is debatable (Leucht et al. 2009). High-dose FGAs should certainly be reviewed in schizophrenia patients manifesting depressive symptoms, as they may be a source of extrapyramidal side effects (EPSE) and psychomotor retardation with direct and indirect influence on depressive symptoms, i.e. be conflated with anhedonia or cause low mood by delaying functional recovery (see Box 10.4). A Cochrane review, finding only one suitable study, concluded that there is no evidence of efficacy for lithium on depressive symptoms in schizophrenia (Leucht et al. 2015).

In sum, there is relatively good evidence that antidepressants are effective in treating depression in people with schizophrenia, and large-scale population data also suggest that this combination does not cause a significant increase in ad-verse events. One should also be aware that some antidepressants have pharma-cokinetic interactions with certain antipsychotics and dose alterations might be required (e.g. fluvoxamine increases the serum levels of clozapine). Also consid-eration should be given to potential cumulative side effects of combinations of antidepressants and antipsychotics. Examples include weight gain with mirtazapine and sexual dysfunction with SSRIs and SNRIs.

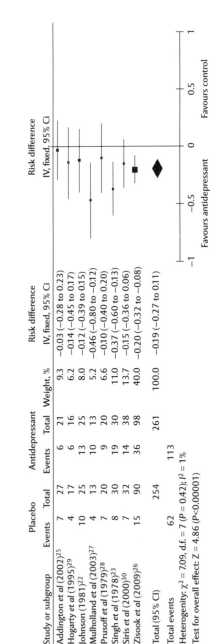

Study or subgroup	Placebo Events	Placebo Total	Antidepressant Events	Antidepressant Total	Weight, %	Risk difference IV, fixed, 95% Ci
Addington et al (2002)[25]	7	27	6	21	9.3	−0.03 (−0.28 to 0.23)
Hogarty et al (1995)[29]	4	17	6	16	6.2	−0.14 (−0.45 to 0.17)
Johnson (1981)[22]	10	25	13	25	8.0	−0.12 (−0.39 to 0.15)
Mulholland et al (2003)[27]	4	13	10	13	5.2	−0.46 (−0.80 to −0.12)
Prusoff et al (1979)[28]	7	20	9	20	6.6	−0.10 (−0.40 to 0.20)
Singh et al (1978)[23]	8	30	19	30	11.0	−0.37 (−0.60 to −0.13)
Siris et al (2000)[30]	7	32	14	38	13.7	−0.15 (−0.36 to 0.06)
Zisook et al (2009)[26]	15	90	36	98	40.0	−0.20 (−0.32 to −0.08)
Total (95% CI)		254		261	100.0	−0.19 (−0.27 to 0.11)
Total events	62		113			

Heterogeneity: $\chi^2 = 7.09$, d.f. = 7 (P = 0.42); $I^2 = 1\%$
Test for overall effect: Z = 4.86 (P<0.00001)

Favours antidepressant   Favours control

Figure 10.1 Forest plot of response (recovery from depression) to adjunctive antidepressant medication in schizophrenia.

> **Box 10.4** Pharmacological and psychosocial management of depression in schizophrenia
>
> - Review antipsychotic dose: exclude EPSE
> - Consider SSRI in individual patient trial
> - Consider antipsychotic dose tapering
> - There is little evidence to support switching antipsychotic, particularly from one SGA to another.
> - Avoid haloperidol
> - There is no evidence for lithium; however, few studies have been conducted
> - CBTp with depression as an outcome may have a modest effect; evidence is limited
> - Interventions aimed at improving psychosocial functioning may be helpful: further trials are needed

Finally, antipsychotic medication and dose should be reviewed in patients presenting with depressive features, as there is evidence to support antidepressant properties in a number of SGAs. Due caution is given about switching, with risk of relapse weighed carefully against any potential mood benefits.

Psychosocial interventions

Taking the evidence from major depressive disorders, the treatment of a depressive episode in schizophrenia ought to benefit from psychological interventions such as CBT, exercise, and structured activity, as well as medication. However, if the evidence for antidepressant medication for the treatment of depression in schizophrenia is less than ideal, that focusing on psychosocial interventions is even more frustrating, with a paucity of high-quality clinical trials. For example, of the published trials of CBTp, none has depression as a primary outcome, and none is sufficiently powered to address the key question as to whether, in the face of depressive comorbidity in schizophrenia, CBT is effective. CBTp has been recommended in guidelines for the treatment of schizophrenia, and the NICE reference a small-to-moderate effect of CBTp on depression (effect size −0.30) (Kuipers et al. 2014).

Some evidence suggests exercise may be effective in treating depression in schizophrenia. Dauwan et al. investigated the effect of exercise in a range of single blind and open trials of exercise interventions in patients with schizophrenia, reporting on a number of outcomes including depression. With a pooled total of 296 patients, exercise reduced depressive symptoms compared to control, with a large pooled effect size of −0.71 (Dauwan et al. 2016). Other treatments in schizophrenia aimed at improving psychosocial functioning, including peer support and vocational interventions, may in theory have potential to reduce isolation and hopelessness, and therefore have secondary effects on comorbid depression, but evidence is limited and what has been published is largely negative (Cook et al. 2012).

Conclusions

Depression is a frequent comorbidity in schizophrenia, is often underrecognized, can be conflated or masked by negative symptoms, and yet has serious consequences for recovery and suicidal behaviour. Specific attention and assessment should be given to patients with incomplete recovery of the possibility of comorbid depression. Effective treatments are likely to include antidepressant medication and potentially CBT and other psychosocial interventions, but the primary research has yet to focus sufficiently on this area of unmet need.

REFERENCES

Addington D, Addington J, Maticka-Tyndale E (1993) Assessing depression in schizophrenia: the Calgary Depression Scale. British Journal of Psychiatry 163: 39–44.

Barnes TR, Drake R, Paton C, et al. (2019) Evidence-based guidelines for the pharmacological treatment of schizophrenia: updated recommendations from the British Association for Psychopharmacology. Journal of Psychopharmacology 34: 3–78.

Birchwood M, Iqbal Z, Upthegrove R (2005) Psychological pathways to depression in schizophrenia: studies in acute psychosis, post psychotic depression and auditory hallucinations. European Archives of Psychiatry and Clinical Neuroscience 255: 202–212.

Buckley PF, Miller BJ, Lehrer DS, Castle DJ (2009) Psychiatric comorbidities and schizophrenia. Schizophrenia Bulletin 35: 383–402.

Busatto GF (2013) Structural and functional neuroimaging studies in major depressive disorder with psychotic features: a critical review. Schizophrenia Bulletin 39: 776–786.

Cleare A, Pariante CM, Young AH, et al. (2015) Evidence-based guidelines for treating depressive disorders with antidepressants: a revision of the 2008 British Association for Psychopharmacology guidelines. Journal of Psychopharmacology 29: 459–525.

Conley RR, Ascher-Svanum H, Zhu B, Faries DE, Kinon BJ (2007) The burden of depressive symptoms in the long-term treatment of patients with schizophrenia. Schizophrenia Research 90: 186–197.

Cook JA, Steigman P, Pickett S, et al. (2012) Randomized controlled trial of peer-led recovery education using Building Recovery of Individual Dreams and Goals through Education and Support (BRIDGES). Schizophrenia Research 136: 36–42.

Cui L, Li M, Deng W, et al. (2011) Overlapping clusters of gray matter deficits in paranoid schizophrenia and psychotic bipolar mania with family history. Neuroscience Letters 489: 94–98.

Dauwan M, Begemann MJ, Heringa SM, Sommer IE (2016) Exercise improves clinical symptoms, quality of life, global functioning, and depression in schizophrenia: a systematic review and meta-analysis. Schizophrenia Bulletin 42: 588–599.

Dutta R, Murray RM, Allardyce J, Jones PB, Boydell J (2011) Early risk factors for suicide in an epidemiological first episode psychosis cohort. Schizophrenia Research 126: 11–19.

Freeman D, Garety PA (2003) Connecting neurosis and psychosis: the direct influence of emotion on delusions and hallucinations. Behaviour Research and Therapy 41: 923–947.

Garety PA, Kuipers E, Fowler D, Freeman D, Bebbington P (2001) A cognitive model of the positive symptoms of psychosis. Psychological Medicine 31: 189–195.

Gregory A, Mallikarjun P, Upthegrove R (2017) Treatment of depression in schizophrenia: systematic review and meta-analysis. The British Journal of Psychiatry 211: 198–204.

Häfner H (2005) Schizophrenia and depression. European Archives of Psychiatry and Clinical Neuroscience 255: 157–158.

Häfner H, Maurer K, Trendler G, An der Heiden W, Schmidt M, Konnecke R (2005) Schizophrenia and depression: challenging the paradigm of two separate diseases—a controlled study of schizophrenia, depression and healthy controls. Schizophrenia Research 77: 11–24.

Hall J (2017) Schizophrenia—an anxiety disorder? British Journal of Psychiatry 211: 262–263.

Helfer B, Samara MT, Huhn M, et al. (2016) Efficacy and safety of antidepressants added to antipsychotics for schizophrenia: a systematic review and meta-analysis. American Journal of Psychiatry 173: 876–886.

International Schizophrenia Consortium (2009) Common polygenic variation contributes to risk of schizophrenia that overlaps with bipolar disorder. Nature 460: 748.

Khandaker GM, Pearson RM, Zammit S, Lewis G, Jones PB (2014) Association of serum interleukin 6 and C-reactive protein in childhood with depression and psychosis in young adult life—a population-based longitudinal study. JAMA Psychiatry 71.

Krynicki C, Upthegrove R, Deakin J, Barnes T (2018) The relationship between negative symptoms and depression in schizophrenia: a systematic review. Acta Psychiatrica Scandinavica 137: 380–390.

Kuipers E, Yesufu-Udechuku A, Taylor C, Kendall T (2014) Management of psychosis and schizophrenia in adults: summary of updated NICE guidance. BMJ 348: g1173.

Leucht S, Corves C, Arbter D, Engel RR, Li C, Davis JM (2009) Second-generation versus first-generation antipsychotic drugs for schizophrenia: a meta-analysis. The Lancet 373: 31–41.

Leucht S, Helfer B, Dold M, Kissling W, McGrath JJ (2015) Lithium for schizophrenia. Cochrane Database of Systematic Reviews 10: CD003834.

McGinty J, Haque MS, Upthegrove R (2018) Depression during first episode psychosis and subsequent suicide risk: a systematic review and meta-analysis of longitudinal studies. Schizophrenia Research 195: 58–66.

Noto C, Ota VK, Santoro ML, et al. (2015) Effects of depression on the cytokine profile in drug naive first-episode psychosis. Schizophrenia Research 164: 53–58.

Palaniyappan L, Hodgson O, Balain V, Iwabuchi S, Gowland P, Liddle P (2019) Structural covariance and cortical reorganisation in schizophrenia: a MRI-based morphometric study. Psychological Medicine 49: 412–420.

Sandhu A, Ives J, Birchwood M, Upthegrove R (2013) The subjective experience and phenomenology of depression following first episode psychosis: a qualitative study using photo-elicitation. Journal of Affective Disorders 149: 166–174.

Tiihonen J, Suokas JT, Suvisaari JM, Haukka J, Korhonen P (2012) Polypharmacy with antipsychotics, antidepressants, or benzodiazepines and mortality in schizophrenia. Archives of General Psychiatry 69: 476–483.

Upthegrove R, Birchwood M, Ross K, Brunett K, McCollum R, Jones L (2010) The evolution of depression and suicidality in first episode psychosis. Acta Psychiatrica Scandinavica 122: 211–218.

Upthegrove R, Manzanares-Teson N, Barnes NM (2014) Cytokine function in medication-naive first episode psychosis: a systematic review and meta-analysis. Schizophrenia Research 155: 101–108.

Upthegrove R, Marwaha S, Birchwood M (2017) Depression and schizophrenia: cause, consequence, or trans-diagnostic issue? Schizophrenia Bulletin 43: 240–244.

Yung AR, Buckby JA, Cotton SM, et al. (2006) Psychotic-like experiences in nonpsychotic help-seekers: associations with distress, depression, and disability. Schizophrenia Bulletin 32: 352–359.

CHAPTER 10

CHAPTER 11

Understanding and assessing substance use in schizophrenia

> **KEY POINTS**
>
> * Substance use is very common amongst people with schizophrenia.
> * Tobacco and alcohol abuse lead the licit substances.
> * The most common illicit drugs of abuse are cannabis and amphetamines or cocaine.
> * These drugs carry a high burden of psychiatric, medical, and psychosocial problems.
> * Understanding reasons for use at an individual level might assist engagement of the patient in a treatment plan.

The use of substances, be they licit or illicit, is regrettably very common amongst people with schizophrenia. The approach of clinicians needs to encompass a high degree of awareness, but to engage the individual in a non-judgemental and supportive manner. This chapter outlines the size of the problem, the impact on illness course, and the assessment of substance use comorbidity in schizophrenia. Treatment approaches are covered in Chapter 12.

The size of the problem

Use of substances of abuse by people with schizophrenia is very common. The population-based ECA study from the US (Regier et al. 1990) reported a lifetime rate of problematic substance use in 47% of respondents with schizophrenia, compared to 16% of the general population. Using a different design, the Australian Survey of High Impact Psychoses (SHIP) assessed substance use rates amongst 1,825 people with psychotic disorders and documented past year rates of 49% for cannabis abuse/dependence, 32% for stimulants, and 27% for other illicit drugs; daily alcohol use was reported by 25% of respondents (Moore et al. 2012).

In a review of the international literature, Cantor-Graae and colleagues (2001) suggested a mean prevalence rate of around 40–60% for any substance of abuse/dependence (excluding caffeine and nicotine) amongst people with schizophrenia. Of course, rates do differ to some extent across jurisdictions and the pattern of drugs used varies dependent upon availability, cost, and legislation. Box 11.1

Box 11.1 Prevalence rate estimates of various substances of abuse amongst people with schizophrenia

- Cigarettes: 60–90%
- Alcohol: 21–68%
- Cannabis: 17–83%
- Stimulants: 13–32%
- Cocaine: 15–50%
- Hallucinogens: 13–18%

Source: Data from Cantor-Graae, E., Nordstrom, L.G., McNeil, T. F. (2001) Substance abuse in schizophrenia: a review of the literature and a study of correlates in Sweden. *Schizophrenia Research*, 48: 69–82; Khokhar, J.Y., Dwiel, L.L., Henricks, A.M., et al. (2018) The link between schizophrenia and substance use disorder: A unifying hypothesis. *Schizophrenia Research*, 194: 78–85.

shows the range of reported rates. Tobacco is consistently the most widely used drug, whilst cannabis is uniformly the most common 'illicit' drug (note it is legal in some jurisdictions), with amphetamines (mostly as crystal methamphetamine) second in much of South East Asia and Australasia; in the US, cocaine is second. We address each of these most prevalent drugs in turn. Note we exclude caffeine, but acknowledge very high rates of use amongst people with schizophrenia.

Substances of abuse used by people with schizophrenia

Tobacco

Tobacco is the most common of all substances used by people with schizophrenia and is associated with myriad physical health issues including various cancers (notably lung). Tobacco smoking also serves as a cumulative risk factor for overall cardiovascular disease risk. Of interest and concern is that whilst many countries have seen a dramatic reduction in cigarette smoking in recent decades in response to public health campaigns and higher cost, people with schizophrenia still smoke at a very high rate. There is also emerging evidence that cigarette smoking is a cumulative causal factor in schizophrenia (Scott et al. 2019).

Theories as to why there are such high smoking rates amongst people with schizophrenia include social affiliation and oral gratification, as well as neurobiological reward and amelioration of withdrawal effects. For a full discussion of smoking and schizophrenia the reader is referred to Chapter 5 of the companion volume in this series, *Physical Health and Schizophrenia* (Castle et al. 2017).

Alcohol

Alcohol is a socially sanctioned drug in most parts of the world. It is also strongly advertised and freely available at many social events. Given the social exclusion of many people with schizophrenia and the high rates of social anxiety (see Chapter 7),

Box 11.2 Potential impacts of excessive alcohol use

Medical
- Obesity and increased cardiovascular risk
- Increased rates of various cancers
- Hepatic, including cirrhosis, cancer
- Head injury
- Withdrawal delirium
- Wernicke's encephalopathy
- Seizures

Psychiatric
- Depression
- Anxiety
- Suicidality
- Cognitive problems (Korsakoff's syndrome, alcoholic dementia)
- Alcoholic hallucinosis
- Pathological jealousy

Psychosocial
- Cost implications for people on low income
- Violence
- Domestic disharmony
- Drunk driving and public order offences
- Other forensic implications

use of alcohol is common amongst this group. The medical, psychiatric, and psychosocial impacts of alcohol abuse are well described (see Box 11.2). People with schizophrenia are arguably at particular risk for a number of these adverse outcomes and it is also recognized that their overall physical health is generally poor and their healthcare suboptimal. Thus, alcohol can be an important added risk factor for early death. There are also implications of alcohol use in people on prescribed psychotropic drugs, as side effects may be exacerbated.

Cannabis

Cannabis use amongst people with schizophrenia has come under particular scrutiny over the last decade, in part because cannabis is becoming more and more potent in terms of its psychotomimetic properties. Thus, the proportion of the main psychotomimetic chemical in the cannabis plant, delta -9-tetrahydrocannabinol, is much higher in modern strains of the plant product, whilst the level of cannabidiol (CBD), which has potential antipsychotic effects, has reduced. The impact of this has been shown in studies that have demonstrated more detrimental impact of high-potency cannabis (known as 'skunk') in people with schizophrenia (Di Forti et al. 2009). Also, legalization (or at least decriminalization) of cannabis in many

> **Box 11.3** Psychiatric and neuropsychiatric effects of cannabis
>
> - Prolongation of the sense of the passage of time
> - Depersonalization/derealization
> - Anxiety: mostly anxiolytic, but can precipitate panic in vulnerable individuals
> - Mood effects: intoxication often results in mirthful laughter; association with depression mostly 'reverse causality'; can result in manic-like episodes in vulnerable individuals
> - Psychosis: transient paranoid ideation and referential thinking
> - Cognitive effects: short-term impairment of concentration and fine motor control; long-term heavy use associated with subacute encephalopathy ('amotivational syndrome'); early heavy use can have (mild) enduring cognitive effects
> - Sleep: users often describe hypnotic effects being a reason for use
> - Appetite often stimulated ('munchies')

jurisdictions, as well as the promotion of medicinal cannabis have led to renewed interest in the compound.

The psychiatric and neuropsychiatric effects of cannabis are well described (Box 11.3). It is fair to say that most of these effects are relatively mild compared to many other drugs, and some of the associations are largely due to reverse causality: for example, most of the association with depression is explicable by use of cannabis by people who already have depression, rather than cannabis being the causal factor for the depression. Having said this, there is particular concern about its impact on people with an underlying vulnerability to mental instability, not least those with schizophrenia. Thus, it is well described that cannabis can worsen the course of established schizophrenia and also that it can 'bring forward' the onset of the illness. The latter has particular implications for young people, as an earlier onset of schizophrenia results in loss of the opportunity to attain key developmental milestones (educational and social) and this in turn has negative implications for long-term functional recovery.

Another key issue is whether cannabis acts as a causal factor in schizophrenia (Castle, 2013). There is now fairly consistent support for this proposition, with a number of high-quality cohort studies showing that cannabis use in youth adds to the risk of a later schizophrenia diagnosis. Of course, the majority of people who use cannabis at any life stage do not go on to develop schizophrenia, and part of the observed associations are confounded by issues such as socioeconomic status and other drug use. But even factoring in such parameters, it is estimated that some 8–10% of people with schizophrenia could have been 'prevented' from manifesting the illness if they had never used cannabis. One of the important tasks for the field is to refine the cumulative risk factors. A genetic loading for schizophrenia, a propensity to 'subthreshold' psychotic symptoms, and a tendency to have a dramatic psychotic experience whilst taking cannabis ('cannabis-precipitated' psychosis: see Chapter 12) are all fairly obvious factors and should act as warning signs for individuals regarding cannabis use. Specific genetic variants, such as AKT1, have some predictive validity, albeit their individual effects are small. Finally, as cautioned above, high potency THC-rich product is particularly dangerous in terms of psychotomimetic effects.

Stimulant drugs

The association between *amphetamines* and schizophrenia has been long appreciated, notably in countries with high rates of use. A number of different longitudinal patterns have been elucidated, namely (see Voce et al. 2019):

* Episodic psychosis on exposure to amphetamines, but with full return to premorbid functioning between episodes
* Repeated episodes with some inter-morbid deficits, including in social and vocational functioning
* Repeated episodes associated with a decline in overall functioning and the evolution of negative symptoms and cognitive deficits which emulates poor-prognosis schizophrenia.

Perhaps the most concerning of the amphetamine class of drugs is the crystalline form of methamphetamine ('crystal meth' or 'ice'), which is a high-potency form of drug which is readily available at low cost in many countries. It is usually smoked or injected, resulting in an almost immediate 'rush' followed by a withdrawal state associated with depressed mood, irritability and craving. It is thus a highly addictive substance.

Amphetamines result in a massive increase in the brain of the neurotransmitters adrenaline, serotonin, and dopamine. The impact of these drugs on the mental state is dramatic and there is a strong association with psychotic symptoms, arousal and violence. These factors are arguably even more dramatic in people with schizophrenia. There are also many acute and longer-term medical complications of methamphetamine use, as outlined in Box 11.4.

Cocaine is a common drug of abuse in the US and rates of use amongst people with schizophrenia are some three to four times the general population rate.

Impact of drugs of abuse on the longitudinal course of schizophrenia

There is a wealth of evidence affirming that drugs of abuse have a negative impact on the trajectory of schizophrenia. This is over and above the damage to physical health that has been outlined above. Of course, the different types of drugs have differential effects on rates of relapse for schizophrenia, and those most likely to result in psychotic relapse are those that increase activity in the dopaminergic

Box 11.4 Short- and long-term psychiatric and medical effects of methamphetamine in schizophrenia

Short-term:
- Severe psychotic episodes with profound motor drive, arousal, and aggression
- Post-high depression
- Craving
- Insomnia
- Hypertension, stroke, aortic dissection
- Serotonin syndrome

Longer-term:
- Psychotic relapses and a 'deficit'-type state
- High rates of dependence
- Perturbations of mood
- Anxiety symptoms
- Insomnia
- Cognitive dysfunction
- Poor dentition
- Skin excoriation
- Cardiomyopathy
- Blood-borne viruses

system. Thus, cannabis has a clear effect in this regard, as do the stimulants such as the amphetamines: the latter are particularly potent and psychosis associated with their use can be very florid and associated with aggression and all the negative impacts this carries for the individual, their families, and people trying to help them. Furthermore, as people experience more and more relapses, their chances of returning to good inter-episode functioning is reduced, and their cognitive functioning is also affected adversely. This downward spiral has far-reaching social consequences for the individual, including loss of work, poverty and social isolation. This is summarized in Box 11.5.

Theories regarding high rates of comorbidity

There have been many attempts to explain the high co-occurrence of substance abuse amongst people with schizophrenia. Green and colleagues (2007) reviewed the literature and proposed a number of explanatory models, as summarized in Box 11.6. Of course, these models are not mutually exclusive. Khokhar et al. (2018) put forward a 'unifying hypothesis', encompassing genetic factors or early environmental insult leading to a dysfunctional mesocorticolimbic system, leaving the individual vulnerable to the use of substances even prior to the manifestation

Box 11.5 Negative impact of drugs of abuse on people with schizophrenia

* Precipitation of psychotic relapse
* Enduring psychotic symptoms
* Accumulating negative symptoms
* Cognitive dysfunction
* Increased rates of emergency department attendance and hospitalization
* High rates of use of restrictive interventions including restraint, seclusion and forced parenteral medication
* Non-adherence to prescribed medications
* Violence
* Domestic violence and estrangement from family
* Children being taken into care
* Criminality
* Poverty
* Prostitution
* Increased rates of blood-borne viruses
* Increased rates of sexually transmitted diseases
* Accidental injury
* Suicide and self-harm
* Early mortality

Source: Data from Smith, J., Hucker, S. (1994) Schizophrenia and substance use disorder. *British Journal of Psychiatry*, 165: 13–21; Lubman, D.I., Sundram, S. (2003) Substance misuse in patients with schizophrenia: a primary care guide. *Medical Journal of Australia*, 178: S71–S75; Unadkat, A., Subasinghe, S., Harvey, R., Castle, D.J. (2019) Methamphetamine use in patients presenting to emergency departments and psychiatric inpatient facilities: what are the service implication? *Australasian Psychiatry*, 27: 14–17.

of psychosis, and also serving as a risk factor for the manifestation of psychotic symptoms as well as to ongoing use of substances. These authors conclude that the field needs to address brain circuitry underpinning psychosis and substance abuse to further advance our understanding of the interaction between these sets of symptoms and associated behaviours.

Self-reported reasons for use

In understanding substance use amongst people with schizophrenia at an individual level, it has been proposed that people with schizophrenia who use drugs do so as a means of 'self-medicating' their psychotic symptoms or associated features such as depression, anxiety and insomnia. To some extent this is true, but the picture is complex. Thus, a study by Spencer et al. (2002) of 69 people with schizophrenia who habitually abused drugs (mostly cannabis)

Box 11.6 Theories regarding comorbidity between schizophrenia and substance abuse

- *Diathesis-stress model*: underlying neurobiological vulnerability with substance use as a 'second hit' leading to the manifestation of schizophrenia
- *Cumulative risk factor model*: cumulative factors associated with schizophrenia (cognitive dysfunction, vocational and social impairment) leaves them vulnerable to substance use
- *Self-medication hypothesis*: use of substance to alleviate symptoms or side effects of medication
- *Primary addiction model*: schizophrenia and substance use disorder driven by deficits in overlapping neural circuitry

Source: Data from Green, A.I., Drake, R.E., Brunette, M.F., Noordsy, D.L. (2007) Schizophrenia and co-occurring substance use disorder. *American Journal of Psychiatry*, 164: 402–408; Khokhar, J.Y., Dwiel, L.L., Henricks, A.M., et al. (2018) The link between schizophrenia and substance use disorder: A unifying hypothesis. *Schizophrenia Research*, 194: 78–85.

---

reported that the substance use was driven by a number of factors, as shown in Box 11.7. By far the most powerful explanatory factor was 'coping with unpleasant affect' (explaining 37% of the variance), followed by 'enhancement' (10%) and 'conformity and acceptance' (8%). Very few people endorsed items relating to positive psychotic symptoms or dealing with side effects of prescribed medication (6% of the variance). Thus, if there is a 'self-medication' effect, it is predominantly to try to ameliorate negative or non-specific anxiety/depressive symptoms.

The importance of understanding reasons for use at an individual level lies not just in the understanding of mechanisms, but can inform a useful dialogue with the individual about other strategies (including prescribed medications) that could be used to ameliorate the target symptoms (e.g. dealing with insomnia through sleep hygiene and judicious use of prescribed hypnotics). It also opens up a broader therapeutic discussion which can be couched in terms of understanding and assisting, rather than judging and blaming. This is expanded upon in Chapter 12.

Conclusions

Substance use is very common amongst people with schizophrenia. Tobacco and alcohol abuse lead the licit substances, whilst the most common illicit drugs of abuse are cannabis and amphetamines or cocaine (depending upon the particular jurisdiction). These drugs carry a high burden of psychiatric, medical and psychosocial problems. Understanding reasons for use at an individual level might assist engagement of the patient in a treatment plan.

Box 11.7 Reasons for use of illicit drugs amongst people with schizophrenia

Coping with unpleasant affect
- Helps with feelings of nervousness
- Helps with feelings of depression
- Helps forget worries
- Helps to feel motivated
- Helps sleep
- Helps concentration
- Helps feelings of self-confidence
- Helps relieve boredom
- Helps decrease restlessness
- Helps to slow down racing thoughts

Enhancement
- Makes one feel good
- Because it is what most friends do
- It is fun
- To get high
- Makes one more sociable
- A way to celebrate
- A way to relax

Conformity and acceptance
- So one won't feel left out
- To be liked
- To help talk to others
- To be sociable
- To be part of a group

Relief of positive symptoms and side effects
- To get away from the voices
- To reduce medication side effects
- Pressure from friends
- To feel less paranoid

Adapted with permission from Spencer, C., Castle, D.J., Michie, P.T. Motivations that maintain substance use among individuals with psychotic disorders. *Schizophrenia Bulletin*, 28: 233–247. Copyright © 2020 Maryland Psychiatric Research Center and Oxford University Press.

REFERENCES

Cantor-Graae E, Nordstrom LG, McNeil TF (2001) Substance abuse in schizophrenia: a review of the literature and a study of correlates in Sweden. Schizophrenia Research 48: 69–82.

Castle D (2013) Cannabis and psychosis: what causes what? F1000 Medicine Reports doi: 10.3410/M5-1 F1000 Med Rep 5:1.

Castle DJ, Buckley PF, Gaughran FP (2017) Physical health and schizophrenia. Oxford: Oxford University Press.

Di Forti M, Morgan C, Dazzan C, et al. (2009) High-potency cannabis and the risk of psychosis. British Journal of Psychiatry 195: 488–491.

Green AI, Drake RE, Brunette MF, Noordsy DL (2007) Schizophrenia and co-occurring substance use disorder. American Journal of Psychiatry 164: 402–408.

Khokhar JY, Dwiel LL, Henricks AM, et al. (2018) The link between schizophrenia and substance use disorder: a unifying hypothesis. Schizophrenia Research 194: 78–85.

Lubman DI, Sundram S (2003) Substance misuse in patients with schizophrenia: a primary care guide. Medical Journal of Australia 178: S71–S75.

Moore E, Mancuso SG, Slade T, et al. (2012) The impact of alcohol and illicit drugs on people with psychosis: the second Australian national survey of psychosis. Australian and New Zealand Journal of Psychiatry 46: 864–878.

Smith J, Hucker S (1994) Schizophrenia and substance use disorder. British Journal of Psychiatry 165: 13–21.

Spencer C, Castle DJ, Michie PT (2002) Motivations that maintain substance use among individuals with psychotic disorders. Schizophrenia Bulletin 28: 233–247.

Unadkat A, Subasinghe S, Harvey R, Castle DJ (2019) Methamphetamine use in patients presenting to emergency departments and psychiatric inpatient facilities: what are the service implications? Australasian Psychiatry 27: 14–17.

CHAPTER 12

Assessment and management of substance abuse comorbidity in people with schizophrenia

KEY POINTS

* Substance abuse and dependence are common amongst people with schizophrenia.
* Assessment requires a careful delineation of drug use effects vs. psychotic symptoms. Motivational interviewing (MI) techniques can be usefully deployed in people with schizophrenia who also abuse substances.
* An integrated framework is preferred for treatment delivery.
* Specific psychological and pharmacological strategies should be considered and tailored to the individual.
* Attention should also be given to adherence with antipsychotic medications.
* Long-acting injectable forms of antipsychotics should be considered.
* Clozapine might have a particular role in people with schizophrenia and substance abuse.

One of the major difficulties in assessing the impact of substances of abuse in people with schizophrenia lies in differentiating the effects of the substance from the core symptoms of schizophrenia. This is critical as it informs treatment. The next challenge is to engage the individual in a discussion about the impact of the substance of abuse on their physical and mental health and to motivate them to address their substance use. This chapter provides a framework for evaluation and engagement as well as outlining treatment options to assist people with schizophrenia and substance abuse comorbidity.

Differentiating substance-induced psychotic symptoms from schizophrenia

It is important to be clear about semantics. All too often clinicians talk of 'drug-induced psychosis' in someone who clearly has an underlying psychotic illness such as schizophrenia, but in whom there is a temporal association between an exposure to a substance of abuse and the manifestation of psychotic symptoms.

> **Box 12.1** Clinical pointers differentiating schizophrenia from drug-induced psychosis
>
> * Psychotic symptoms precede substance use
> * Psychotic symptoms persist despite abstinence (a one-month cut-off is usually applied)
> * Psychotic symptoms manifest even when substances are not used
> * The manifest psychotic symptoms are not of a form or content usually seen in conjunction with the particular substance
> * There is a personal past history of schizophrenia
> * There is a family history of schizophrenia
>
> Adapted with permission from Lubman, D.I., Sundram, S. Substance misuse in patients with schizophrenia: A primary care guide. *Medical Journal of Australia*, 178: S71–75. Copyright © 2003 Wiley. Data from Woody, G., Schuckit, M., Weinrieb, R., Yu, E. A review of the substance use disorders section of the DSM-IV. *Psychiatr Clin North Am*, 1993; 16: 21–32.

In such individuals the preferred term is 'drug-precipitated psychosis', acknowledging the underlying psychotic predisposition. 'Drug-induced psychosis' should, in our view, be applied to those drug-induced toxidromes in which psychotic symptoms are present but which abate over a short period (usually 24–48 hours, depending upon the half-life of the particular drug) and there is no residuum.

It is not always easy to tease out the effects of a substance on mental state if the person continues to use the drug in question. A very careful longitudinal history with collateral, especially mapping periods of drug use and abstinence, and concomitant impact of mental state is critical. If possible, observation of the individual whilst not under the influence of drugs allows one to establish their 'baseline' mental state and functioning. Of course, one needs to manage withdrawal effects (see below) and in long-term users of long-half-life drugs such as cannabis to give sufficient time for the drug to clear the brain (this can take up to a month in the case of cannabis).

There are a number of useful clinical pointers regarding the differentiation of drug-induced psychoses from schizophrenia. These are summarized in Box 12.1.

Treatment frameworks

Many commentators have pointed out the relative dearth of good-quality controlled trial evidence to support specific interventions for people with schizophrenia and substance abuse. In part this is due to the inherent difficulties in engaging and retaining such individuals in clinical trials, and also speaks to the complexity of the clinical picture, with severe psychotic symptoms intersecting with high volumes of use of (often) multiple drugs, and with other psychiatric and medical morbidities adding to the burden (see Chapter 12).

Box 12.2 Overarching models of service delivery for people with schizophrenia and substance abuse

- *Sequential*: dealing with one disorder, then dealing with the other: this involves different service settings and different clinicians
- *Parallel*: each set of problems being dealt with at the same time, but independently and by different clinicians in separate services, often using different models of care
- *Integrated*: this is the preferred model, whereby both sets of problems are dealt with at the same time by clinicians who are skilled in models that address both problems coherently

Adapted with permission from Lubman, D. I., King, J. A., Castle, D. J. (2010) Treating comorbid substance use in schizophrenia. *International Review of Psychiatry*, 22: 191–201.

This lack of empirical data is compounded by treatment service structures that do not lend themselves to dealing with multiple problems simultaneously. In particular, drug and alcohol and mental health services are often under discrete governance and funding models and this leads all too often to either sequential or parallel care for people with schizophrenia who have drug use problems (see Box 12.2). Lubman and colleagues (2010) suggest that this might be adequate for people with milder forms of disorder, but it does not adequately meet the needs of those with severe and protracted disorders, where an integrated model is preferred. Such a model allows a comprehensive approach in a single service setting and ensures that each set of problems is addressed, along with acknowledgement of the interactions between them. Also, as Horsfall et al. (2009) point out, it is important to address basic issues such as finances and housing as part of a treatment plan.

Motivational interviewing

Motivational interviewing (MI) is employed widely in the drug and alcohol sector, as part of an engagement process and setting up a treatment plan. We consider it here in some detail separately from other psychosocial interventions, as we see it as a component part of a comprehensive treatment plan, rather than a complete treatment in itself. Other psychosocial treatments are discussed below. The idea of MI is to map the 'stage of change' of the individual and to have a discussion that serves to move them along the continuum towards acceptance of treatment (see Box 12.3). Baker et al. (2002) suggested that even very brief 'opportunistic' interventions can be successful, but their own study of 160 psychiatric inpatients with drug and alcohol problems (alcohol, cannabis and amphetamines) failed to show any benefit from a 30- to 60-minute manualized MI session in terms of engagement with a substance abuse specialist

Box 12.3 Principles of MI techniques tailored to stage of change

Precontemplation: provide education about current levels of substance use and enable a discussion about problems associated with current level and pattern of use, as well as other risks such as those associated with injecting drug use

Contemplation: whilst acknowledging the patient's resistance to change, discuss the pros and cons of both continuing to use and cutting down or ceasing use; offer specific discussion about the impact of the substance on psychiatric symptoms; also address antipsychotic medications and adherence issues

Preparation: work with the patient to scope the potential change strategies and provide information about such strategies

Action: work with the patient to put a change plan into action; cognitive behavioural coping skills can be particularly helpful

Maintenance: underscore the new skills learnt and emphasize using these skills both to maintain gains and deal with situations in which there is a high risk of relapse

Relapse: continue to emphasize what strategies have been effective in the past, and maintain belief in being able to get back on track after a relapse

Source: Data from Baker, A., Lewin, T., Reichler, H., et al (2002) Motivational interviewing among psychiatric in-patients with substance use disorders. *Acta Psychiatrica Scandinavica*, 106: 233–240; Lubman, D.I., Sundram, S. (2003) Substance misuse in patients with schizophrenia: A primary care guide. *Medical Journal of Australia*, 178: S71–75.

unit. Posited reasons for this disappointing outcome include the severity of the clinical state and the lack of ability to address the substance use issue within the mental health service. This reinforces the virtue of integrated service arrangements, as detailed above. Multisession MI interventions have been shown to have efficacy for some people, albeit the studies are not consistent (see Drake et al. 2008). It should also be emphasized that it often takes a number of 'cycles' of MI before traction is effected. Linking with cognitive behavioural and other approaches can enhance outcomes, as outlined below.

Psychosocial treatments

Drake and colleagues (2008) conducted a useful systematic review of psychosocial treatments for people with substance use and severe mental illness. They endorse the integrated approach outlined above and emphasize the benefits in terms of both access and individualization of care. The more recent Canadian Guidelines (Crockford and Addington 2017) are largely synergistic with these findings and suggestions and add the importance of involving families (where appropriate) in treatment planning and execution. Box 12.4 summarizes the

> **Box 12.4** Summary of psychosocial interventions for substance use comorbidity in people with schizophrenia
>
> • Individual counselling
> • Group counselling
> • Family interventions
> • Case management
> • Residential treatment
> • Intensive outpatient rehabilitation
> • Contingency management
> • Legal intervention
>
> Adapted with permission from Drake, R.E., O'Neal, E.L., Wallach, M.A. A systematic review of psychosocial research on psychosocial interventions for people with co-occurring severe mental and substance use disorders. *Journal of Substance Abuse Treatment*, 34: 123–138. Copyright (c) 2008 Elsevier.

interventions; the text follows Drake et al. (2008), to which article the reader is referred for original references.

Individual counselling includes the MI studies reviewed above, as well as MI linked to CBT. Perhaps the most impressive of these is the long-term study of Barrowclough et al. (2001) in that they incorporated MI, CBT, and a family intervention component delivered over a period of 9 months. There were initial benefits on some measures, but mostly they were not sustained at 18 months.

Group counselling interventions, mostly using CBT strategies, have been fairly consistent in terms of positive outcomes for substance use as well as broader parameters including mental health symptoms. An illustrative example is that of James et al. (2004).

Family interventions specifically addressing people with schizophrenia who have substance use problems have been the subject of very few comprehensive clinical trials. The long-term intervention of Barrowclough et al. (2001)—described above—included a family component, but it is difficult to tease out the efficacy or otherwise of that specific element of what was a comprehensive set of interventions. Despite this lack of empirical data, the Canadian Guidelines (Crockford and Addington 2017) have three specific recommendations regarding family members, namely:

• Encourage families to be involved and to support recovery
• Offer family members an assessment of their own health and social needs
• Provide appropriate information to family members.

Case management refers to intensive multidisciplinary team interventions that include outreach. A mix of different methods have been used to explore efficacy, with mixed results, suggesting that they need to ensure they employ specific strategies for both the mental health and substance use problems to be effective. Irrespective, intensive case management can provide a useful 'holding environment' for the patient and allow other more specific work to be done.

Residential treatments are those offered in full-time residential settings, usually over 6–12 months. Programs offered vary across settings. The evidence suggests that longer-term placements are generally more effective than shorter-term.

Intensive outpatient rehabilitation is equivalent to day programmes, offering intensive programmes on several days of the week (some offer evening sessions). One of the problems is high attrition rates.

Contingency management involves the provision of incentives (or disincentives) contingent upon drug use status. The aim is to modify drug use behaviours. Results of studies to date are encouraging, but it can be difficult to set such services up, and some jurisdictions have an ethical objection to such 'incentivization'.

Legal interventions encompass a variety of mandated treatment models, including prison diversion schemes. Such services can effect enhanced attendance for treatment, but whether they have long-term benefits for substance use is not clearly determined.

Pharmacological interventions

Pharmacological interventions for substance use problems in schizophrenia are employed in different contexts with different strategic intentions. In withdrawal states, the intent is to ensure as safe and undistressing a withdrawal as possible. In drug-induced toxidromes and drug-precipitated psychoses, the aim is to settle the person's aroused mental state as quickly and safely as possible to avoid danger to self, others, or property. In the maintenance phase, the aim is to reduce the likelihood of relapse. All these phases require exquisite attention to the particulars of the individual and interventions need to be nuanced to the specific drug of abuse. Also, consideration needs to be given to the prescribed drugs the individual is taking, as there might be interaction effects. Attention needs to be given to choice of, and adherence issues with, antipsychotic medications.

Withdrawal

Withdrawal states differ across drugs of abuse, dependent, inter alia, upon their pharmacodynamics and their excretion half-life, as well as being influenced by the duration of use and the dose of the particular agent. Thus, in chronic heavy users, drugs such as alcohol can have dramatic and dangerous withdrawal states, whilst with cannabis—which is highly lipophilic and takes a long time to be excreted— the withdrawal state, whilst unpleasant, is usually more benign.

Stabilizing the patient medically is an imperative. Thiamine replacement and other established measures are required in alcohol withdrawal states. Benzodiazepines such as diazepam are often used to treat withdrawal states and can be safely used in people with schizophrenia, with the caveat that this group might be particularly vulnerable to respiratory depression consequent upon high rates of obesity and poor respiratory health.

Treating toxidromes and drug-precipitated psychotic states

The immediate treatment of an individual with schizophrenia presenting with a psychotic episode in the context of substance use needs to be tailored to the drug of abuse as well as the level of arousal. Aggression is common in association with stimulants and needs specific management. In terms of medications, oral antipsychotics might be either refused by the patient or simply not be sufficiently fast-acting. In such situations, parenteral (intramuscular or intravenous) administration might be required; adjunctive benzodiazepines can be considered (Galletly et al. 2016). Care needs to be taken to monitor the patient's physical status, including dystonias (laryngeal dystonias can be fatal), respiration (benzodiazepines can suppress the respiratory centre) and cardiac function (a number of antipsychotics can prolong the corrected QT interval (QTc) and result in dysrhythmias). Figure 12.1 provides an algorithm for use in the management of acute psychotic states in people with psychotic disorders.

Pharmacological approaches to establishing and maintaining abstinence

Smoking

There is a well-established set of medications that assist smokers in quitting, as shown in Table 12.1. These agents can be effective for smokers with schizophrenia, but some have potential psychiatric side effects, which makes their use in people with schizophrenia potentially troublesome. Bupropion can cause maniform episodes in vulnerable individuals, but is usually safe in people with schizophrenia. The most effective of the smoking cessation agents is the partial nicotinic agonist varenicline. Initial concerns about its use in people with mental illness have largely been allayed by the large-scale Evaluating Adverse Events in a Global Smoking Cessation Study (EAGLES) trial, in which 3,984 smokers without a prior mental illness and 4,050 smokers with a prior mental illness (10% psychotic disorders) were randomized to nicotine replacement therapy, bupropion, varenicline, or placebo (Anthenelli et al. 2019). Neuropsychiatric adverse events (NPSAEs) of a moderate or severe level were experienced by 2.1% of those without a prior psychiatric history and 5.9% with such a history, but there were no significant differences among the active interventions. Overall, current anxiety and past suicidality predicted NPSAEs, whilst in the mental illness group, predictors were younger age, female sex, history of substance abuse, higher nicotine dependence and greater psychiatric illness severity (Anthenelli et al. 2019). The caveat here is that only people with stable psychiatric symptoms were included, meaning that inferences for people with unstable psychotic symptoms in particular cannot be drawn.

Our advice is that people with schizophrenia who smoke should be offered the full range of psychological and pharmacotherapy interventions, but they should be

STEP 1 - (Arousal level 2-3)

Mildly aroused, pacing, still willing to talk reasonably.
Moderately aroused, agitated, becoming more vocal, unreasonable or hostile.

ORAL

Lorazepam (peak effect at 1-3 hrs): 1 to 2 mg, repeated every 2-6 hrs to a maximum of 10 mg in 24 hrs

OR

Olanzapine (peak effect at 1-3 hrs): 5-10 mg repeated if necessary every 2 hrs to a maximum of 30 mg in 24 hrs.

Review after 30-60 minutes, repeat if necessary

If still ineffective, consider Step 2

In smokers, consider NRT where possible (REGULAR patch ± PRN inhaler or lozenges)

PRECAUTIONS:

Lower doses should be considered in the elderly, patients with low body weight, dehydration or no previous exposure to antipsychotic medication.

Vigilant monitoring for signs of: airway obstruction, respiratory depression and hypotension every 15 minutes for 90 minutes during the post-medication period and hourly thereafter.

Monitor ECG, FBE, U&E, Mg, CK & troponin if using high doses of antipsychotics or Cloplxol Acuphase®.

Assess and manage DVT risk—consider DVT prophylaxis

STEP 2 - (Arousal level 3-4)

Moderately aroused, agitated, becoming more vocal, unreasonable and hostile.
Highly aroused, possibly distressed and fearful.

ORAL

Olanzapine (peak effect at 6 hrs): 10-20 mg repeated if necessary every 2-6 hrs up to a maximum of 30 mg in 24 hrs.

PLUS

Lorazepam (peak effect at 1-3hrs): 1 to 2 mg, repeated every 2-6 hrs, up to a maximum of 10 mg in 24 hrs.

Review after 30-60 minutes, repeat if necessary.

If still ineffective, consider Step 3

Consider what sensory interventions may be appropriate

Create opportunity and environment for patient to express fears, frustration, anger, etc. (Ventilation)

Explore with patient what interventions/solutions would assist them to gain control (Redirection)

Assess "time out" opportunity for patient to regain control (5-15 mins duration) (Time Out)

Post Traumatic Event Support should be offered to:

Provide the opportunity for anyone involved in an aggressive incident, or restrictive practice to voice their feelings, opinions and reactions about their experience.

STEP 3 - (Arousal level 4-5)

Refusing oral medication, moderately aroused, agitated, becoming more vocal, unreasonable and hostile.
Highly aroused, distressed and fearful; violent toward self, others or property.

INTRAMUSCULAR

1st Line:
Olanzapine (peak effect at 15-45 mins):
10 mg repeated if necessary every 2 hrs to a maximum of 30 mg in 24 hrs.

2nd Line: (preferred option for stimulant toxicity)
Droperidol (Onset of action 3-10 mins):
2.5 to 10 mg every 20 minutes to a maximum of 20 mg in 24 hrs (where possible obtain an ECG).

*Clonazepam (peak effect at 3 hrs): if tranquillisation not achieved, this can be used in addition to the above options, BUT not at the same time. A gap of 1 hr is required between Clonazepam & Droperidol IMI or 2 hrs between Clonazepam & Olanzapine IMI.
1-2 mg may repeat after 2 hrs, then every 4 hrs up to 4 mg in 24 hrs

Note: Cloplxol A cuphase® might be used as per separate protocol, as a treatment regimen (NOT 'prn')
2mg dose clonazepam can be diluted in 1 ml diluent

ALERTS:

! Extrapyramidal side effects must be assessed and treated.

! Anticholinergic agents NOT to be used routinely but 'as required' (PRN); Benztropine 2 mg IMI may be used for acute dystonias (Max 6 mg/24 hrs).

! Clonazepam has a long half-life of 3-40 hours; therefore it can accumulate with repeated administration increasing risk of over-sedation and respiratory depression

NOTE: these guidelines are reflective of the local Australian context; other jurisdictions might have other preferred medications (eg. lorazepam is the preferred IM benzodiazepine but is not universally available)

Figure 12.1 Guidelines for pharmacological management of acute behavioural disturbance in psychosis.

Reproduced from Barnes, C.W., Alderton, D., Castle, D. The development of clinical guidelines for the use of Zuclopenthixol acetate. Australasian Psychiatry, 10: 54–58. Copyright © 2002. © SAGE Publications.

Table 12.1 Approved drugs for treating nicotine dependence

Drug	Recommended dose	Course of treatment	Common adverse effects	
Nicotine replacement therapies (NRT)				**Directions for use**
Nicotine patch 24 h: 21 mg, 14 mg1 7mg 16 h: 25 mg, 10 mg	Start with full-strength patch if ≥ 10 cigs/day	12 weeks	Insomnia, disturbed dreams (24-h patch) Skin irritation	Apply in the morning to upper arm, chest, or back and rotate application site daily
Nicotine mouth spray: 1 mg per spray	1–2 sprays every 30–60 minutes Maximum 4 sprays/h or 64 sprays/day	12 weeks	Mouth/throat irritation, nausea, dyspepsia, headache, hiccups	Fast-acting craving relief. Spray under tongue or onto inside of cheek
Nicotine oral strips: 2.5 mg	Initially 1 strip every 1–2 h, up to 15/day	12 weeks	Nausea, throat irritation, hiccups, headache	Fast-acting craving relief for less-dependent smokers. Place on tongue and apply to palate: dissolves in 2–3 minutes
Nicotine lozenges: 2 mg, 4 mg	9–15/day	12 weeks	Nausea, hiccups, heartburn, flatulence	Allow to dissolve in the mouth over 20–30 minutes, moving around from time to time
Nicotine mini lozenges: 1.5 mg, 4 mg	1.5 mg: 9–20 times/day 4 mg: 9–15/day	12 weeks	Nausea, hiccups, heartburn, flatulence	Allow to dissolve in the mouth over 10–15 minutes, moving around from time to time
Nicotine gum: 2 mg, 4 mg	2 mg: 8–20/day 4 mg: 4–10/day. Use 4 mg if TTFC ≤ 30 minutes	12 weeks	Hiccups, nausea, jaw discomfort, mouth/throat irritation	Instruct patients on 'park and chew' technique[a]. Avoid in people with dentures

continued >

Table 12.1 Continued

Drug	Recommended dose	Course of treatment	Common adverse effects	
Nicotine inhalator: 15 mg per cartridge	3–6 cartridges/ day	12 weeks	Cough, mouth/throat irritation, nausea	Frequent shallow puffs. Satisfies hand-to-mouth habit
Non-nicotine tablets				**Comments**
Varenicline: 0.5 mg, 1 mg	0.5 mg/day for 3 days, then 0.5 bd for 4 days, then 1 mg bd	12 weeks; optional second course	Nausea, insomnia, disturbed dreams, headache, drowsiness	Most effective monotherapy. Take with a meal to reduce nausea. No known drug interactions. Contraindicated in pregnancy and lactation
Bupropion: 150 mg	150 mg/day for 3 days, then 150 mg bd	9 weeks	Seizure risk 1:1,000, insomnia, headache, dry mouth	Elevated seizure risk. Numerous potential drug interactions. Contraindicated in pregnancy and lactation

TTFC, Time to first cigarette.

ᵃChew gum slowly until peppery taste appears and then place gum in the buccal pouch until taste fades. Chew again until taste appears. Repeat cycle for 30 minutes, then discard. Avoid swallowing nicotine.

Reproduced with permission from Mendelsohn, C. P., Kirby, D. P., Castle, D.J., Smoking and mental illness. An update for psychiatrists. *Australasian Psychiatry*, 23(1): 37–43. Copyright © The Royal Australian and New Zealand College of Psychiatrists 2014.

given extra support and monitoring of mental state especially over the first few weeks of treatment. It must also be borne in mind that smoking cessation can result in increased blood levels of clozapine, olanzapine and haloperidol, and dosage adjustments might be required. For a full discussion of these issues the reader is referred to Chapter 5 of the companion volume in this series, *Physical Health and Schizophrenia* (Castle et al. 2017).

Alcohol

Naltrexone has been shown to be safe and effective as an adjunct to antipsychotic medications in people with schizophrenia who abuse alcohol, but studies are sparse, small, and short-term (Petrakis et al. 2006). Disulfiram has also been used in this clinical scenario, with reductions in alcohol use and improvement in psychotic symptoms (Petrakis et al. 2006). Acamprosate has no current evidence to support use in people with schizophrenia (Crockford and Addington 2017).

Cannabis

There are more negative than positive trials of medications to assist with cannabis use disorder: bupropion, mirtazapine, dronabinol and nabilone have all failed in clinical trials. Crockford and Addington (2017) make no recommendations for specific medications for cannabis abuse in the context of schizophrenia.

Amphetamines

There have been many failed studies of pharmacological treatment for amphetamine users, including sertraline, bupropion, ondansetron and modafinil. Mirtazepine has shown some benefits (Coffin et al. 2020) but has not to our knowledge been tested in amphetamine users with schizophrenia. Trials of substitution with lisdexamphetamine for amphetamine users are in progress, but not in people with schizophrenia, and stimulants carry the propensity to exacerbate psychosis. Thus, no medication can be recommended specifically in this context.

Cocaine

The use of imipramine and desipramine has been explored for cocaine users with schizophrenia, but the quality of the studies was low and results inconsistent. Crockford and Addington (2017) suggest that risks associated with tricyclics and this low evidence base cannot support the use of any specific medications for cocaine users with schizophrenia.

Implications for antipsychotic therapy

Non-adherence to prescribed medications is all too common in any chronic health condition, and people with schizophrenia are particularly prone to not taking their medications as prescribed. The reasons for this are complex and encompass medication side effects, as well as negative beliefs about the role of medications in therapy. These problems are exacerbated in people with schizophrenia who also use illicit drugs (see Chapter 11). Some patients state that side effects of medications make them feel emotionally blunted and this can increase substance use. This effect was arguably more pronounced with the older 'typical' antipsychotic drugs, but there has been little compelling evidence to suggest lower illicit drug use being associated with atypical antipsychotics: apart from clozapine, that is (Green et al. 2002). Clozapine is a unique drug and often is helpful in symptom amelioration in people who have not responded adequately to other antipsychotics. However, its burden of side effects (weight gain, sedation, agranulocytosis, myocarditis, cardiomyopathy) leaves it usually being reserved for people who have proven 'treatment-resistant' schizophrenia. Substance use comorbidity is not usually a major consideration in choosing clozapine, but perhaps it should be, as a number of studies have suggested it reduces the drive to use illicit drugs. For example, Siskind et al. (2017) showed in a large Australian sample of people with psychotic disorders that people on clozapine had lower rates of current substance abuse, albeit their lifetime rates of using such drugs was no different from patients not on clozapine.

Another consideration for clinicians is whether to promote the use of long-acting injectable antipsychotics (LAIs) specifically in people with schizophrenia who abuse drugs. There is intrinsic appeal to this approach, given the often chaotic nature of such individual's lives and the catastrophic effects of frequent psychotic relapses. Unfortunately, the evidence base for use of LAIs in such patients is sparse, reflecting clinical complexity and difficulties with informed consent. But those few studies that have been conducted do suggest benefit for this approach. For example, studies of the depot formulation of the typical antipsychotic flupenthixol have shown particular benefits for reduction of alcohol use (Soyka et al. 2003); and the atypical agent risperidone in long-acting formulation has been shown to be effective in reducing substance use as well as improving psychopathology scores in people with schizophrenia and substance use comorbidity (Rubio et al. 2006). Certainly clinicians and families are mostly relieved that with a depot antipsychotic adherence is assured, allowing more focus on those psychosocial parameters of care outlined above.

Conclusions

Substance abuse and dependence are common amongst people with schizophrenia. Assessment requires a careful delineation of drug use affects vs. psychotic symptoms and also contributing factors to each set of problems. Engagement of the individual can be enhanced through use of a non-judgemental but firm approach: motivational interviewing techniques can be usefully deployed. It is best to deliver care using an integrated framework. Specific psychological and pharmacological strategies should be considered and tailored to the individual. Attention should also be given to adherence with antipsychotic medications, and long-acting injectable forms should be considered. Clozapine might have a particular role in people with schizophrenia and substance abuse.

REFERENCES

Anthenelli RM, Gaffney M, Benowitz NL, et al. (2019) Predictors of neuropsychiatric adverse events with smoking cessation medications in the randomised controlled EAGLES trial. Journal of General Internal Medicine 34: 862–870.

Baker A, Lewin T, Reichler H, et al (2002) Motivational interviewing among psychiatric in-patients with substance use disorders. Acta Psychiatrica Scandinavica 106: 233–240.

Castle DJ, Buckley PF, Gaughran FP (2017) Physical health and schizophrenia. Oxford: Oxford University Press, pp. 39–50.

Coffin PO, Santos G-M, Hern J, et al. (2020) Effects of mirtazapine for methamphetamine use disorder among cisgender men and transgender women who have sex with men: a placebo-controlled randomised clinical trial. JAMA Psychiatry 77: 246–255.

Crockford D, Addington D (2017) Canadian schizophrenia guidelines: schizophrenia and other psychotic disorders with coexisting substance use disorders. Canadian Journal of Psychiatry 62: 624–634.

Drake RE, O'Neal EL, Wallach MA (2008) A systematic review of psychosocial research on psychosocial interventions for people with co-occurring severe mental and substance use disorders. Journal of Substance Abuse Treatment 34: 123–138.

Galletly C, Castle DJ, Dark F, et al (2016) Clinical practice guideline for the management of schizophrenia and related disorders. Australian & New Zealand Journal of Psychiatry 50: 410–472.

Green AI, Salomon MS, Brenner MJ, Rawlins K (2002) Treatment of schizophrenia and comorbid substance use disorder. Current Drug Targets: CNS and Neurological Disorders 1: 129–139.

Horsfall J, Cleary M, Hunt G, Walter G (2009) Psychosocial treatments for people with co-occurring severe mental illness and substance use disorders (dual diagnosis): a review of empirical evidence. Harvard Review of Psychiatry 17: 24–34.

James W, Preston N, Koh G, et al (2004) A group intervention which assists patients with dual diagnosis reduce their drug use: a randomised controlled trial. Psychological Medicine 34: 983–990.

Lubman DI, Sundram S (2003) Substance misuse in patients with schizophrenia: a primary care guide. Medical Journal of Australia 178: S71–S75.

Lubman DI, King JA, Castle DJ (2010) Treating comorbid substance use in schizophrenia. International Review of Psychiatry 22: 191–201.

Petrakis IL, Nich C, Ralevski E (2006) Psychotic spectrum disorders and alcohol abuse: a review of pharmacotherapeutic strategies and a report on the effectiveness of naltrexone and disulfiram. Schizophrenia Bulletin 32: 644–654.

Rubio G, Martinez I, Ponce G, et al (2006) Long-acting injectable risperidone compared with zuclopenthixol in the treatment of schizophrenia with substance abuse comorbidity. Canadian Journal of Psychiatry 51: 531–539.

Siskind D, Harris M, Phillipou A, et al (2017) Clozapine users in Australia: their characteristics and experiences of care based on data from the 2010 national survey of high impact psychosis. Epidemiology and Psychiatric Sciences 26: 325–337.

Soyka M, Aichmuller C, Bardeleben U, et al. (2003) Flupenthixol in relapse prevention in schizophrenics with comorbid alcoholism: results from an open clinical study. European Addiction Research 9: 65–72.

Index

For the benefit of digital users, indexed terms that span two pages (e.g., 52–53) may, on occasion, appear on only one of those pages.

Tables, figures and boxes are indicated by *t*, *f* and *b* following the page number